S E E N

SEEN

A MEMOIR

LEAH ZACCARIA

higgins

PRESS

Published by Higgins Press, Seattle

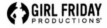

Edited and Designed by Girl Friday Productions
www.girlfridayproductions.com
Editorial: Alexander Rigby, Anna Katz, Valerie
Paquin, Sharon Turner Mulvihill
Cover & Interior Design: Rachel Marek

ISBN (Hardcover): 978-1-7326786-1-3
ISBN (Paperback): 978-1-7326786-0-6
e-ISBN: 978-1-7326786-2-0

First Edition

Printed in the United States of America

For my daughter Alexis Zaccaria.
Thank you for braving this journey with me.

Contents

Introduction

I can hear my dad pounding on the front door. He is screaming for us to let him in. I know he's drunk, and I'm so scared. I don't know what he'll do next. I don't want him to find me if he manages to get inside, so I crawl under the dining room table to hide. It's late, and I'm wearing my Strawberry Shortcake pajamas.

After what feels like hours but is probably just a few minutes, I muster up the courage to crawl back out and grab the phone off the wall, then rush back to my hiding spot, the long, curly cord stretching between me and the wall. I am shivering with fear. With a shaking hand, I dial the number to the restaurant where my mom works as a cocktail waitress. She finally gets on the line.

"Mom," I say, "please come home! Dad is drunk and I'm afraid. Please, Mom. Please! I don't know what to do. Help me."

"I can't leave. If I do I'll lose my job," she says, then hangs up the phone.

———

We all want to be seen. More than that, it is our divine right to be seen.

What I mean by *seen* is to feel loved and accepted, to stand fully in our truths, to be naked in vulnerability, to live in the most authentic way. It is refusing to be what others want or think we should be, and instead being who we are in every facet of our lives.

I believe true freedom lies in being and feeling seen; that through living in truth we can embody love and acceptance of both our own uniqueness and that of others. Then and only then can we fully realize our purpose and serve the world through the gifts we bring.

In order to be fully seen, we have to let untruths die, a lifelong process of letting go and rebirth. This process can be painful, and most of us hide ourselves instead of seeking the truth, out of fear of rejection, judgment, failure, or loss. To come out of hiding takes a great deal of courage, strength, and vulnerability. It is a hero's journey, an adventure into the unknown in the hope of transformation.

I share my story in the following pages because we all go through the same things. None of us are alone—though we may feel lonely at times, we are all facing this together.

Throughout my journey, I have come to the conclusion that the human experience goes through what I call Seen Cycles. The Seen Cycles are the processes by which we try to be seen and, hopefully, are ultimately seen. I call them *cycles* because within each of them, there are patterns that are repeated over and over if we are not transformed. Phases are temporary stages that typically run their course, whereas cycles reoccur unless broken. Cycles take much more effort to move through than phases do.

There are five Seen Cycles: Primal, Struggle, Conform, Transform, and Purpose. The first three cycles—Primal, Struggle, and Conform—are the cycles in which we seek to be seen by sources outside ourselves. The last two cycles—Transform and Purpose—are the cycles in which we seek to see ourselves from within.

I believe that we all go through the first three cycles, that no one is exempt. But we don't all go through the last two cycles. Many of us get stuck in the Conform Cycle, looking externally for validation for the duration of our lives. Getting to the Transform and Purpose Cycles takes great courage and action. It takes effort and the willingness to feel, endure, and commit to growth and exploration.

My mission for this book is to share my journey through these cycles in the hope that you will be able to relate to and apply the lessons I learned to your own life. I hope to inspire and empower you to see yourself and to be fully seen. I hope you will give yourself permission to let some things die for the sake of rebirth. To truly show yourself can make you feel scared and vulnerable. But if you pay enough attention to the brief glimpses you have of your true self, listen to the whispers from your inner knowing, then you will finally see and be seen.

Please note: some names have been changed to protect the guilty and the innocent.

The Primal Cycle

"Don't turn away from what's painful. Examine it. Challenge it."

—*Steven Spielberg*

We can't avoid the Primal Cycle. From day one, we are under the care of another human, whether it's a nuclear family, group of loving adults, or series of sometimes overworked, underpaid caretakers at a children's home or other institution. These early relationships are essential for determining how we will feel seen and be seen. I have a mother and father, so I will share through that lens.

It starts in the womb. Did our mothers want us? Were they able to take care of themselves during pregnancy? Did we share the womb with a sibling? Was there stress? Nourishment? Did our mothers sing to us, dream about us, pray for us? These all are important factors in how we feel, and how we interpret the world.

When we are born, our lifeline is our mother or another caretaker. For the sake of simplicity, I will use feminine pronouns, though a caretaker doesn't have to be female, and hopefully there is more than one. We depend on her to keep us alive. In a perfect world, she feeds us, bathes us, and nurtures us. She is our protector. She keeps us safe from harm.

We seek to love and be loved by her. It is primal and innate. Everything we seek we seek through her, because we do not yet know how to find it for ourselves. If we do not feel seen, accepted, or loved by our mother, if she fails us or abandons us, we will seek protection from other sources. There is no way around it.

Both my mother and father came from big Catholic families. They grew up going to Catholic Mass in their Sunday best and living the Catholic lifestyle. My mom went to an all-girls Catholic high school, and my dad went to an all-boys Catholic high school, both in Spokane, Washington. My mom was beautiful. She had long, flat-ironed blonde hair, blue eyes, and a curvaceous body. My dad was also a looker. He was an all-star football player with muscular legs and a medium build, jet-black hair, and piercing blue eyes. My parents' schools often came together for dances, and that was where they met. When they were both eighteen years old and still in high school, they got pregnant with my sister Holly.

After graduation, they moved to Missoula, Montana, so my dad could study to be a doctor. But two years after Holly was born, I came along, and he dropped out of school and we moved back to Spokane. There my parents bought a house and started working, my dad as a chef and my mom as a waitress.

My parents did not have a lot of money, but they had support from their families. All four of my grandparents were successful professionals, a rarity in that day and age. My maternal grandmother was a communications executive, and my maternal grandfather owned a construction company. My paternal grandmother was a nurse, and my paternal grandfather was a well-known general surgeon. Though my parents had mostly good relationships with their parents, when my mom and dad were kids their parents weren't home a lot, and other family members or nannies had been responsible for most of the childcare. My mom credits her grandmother with raising her, while my dad had various nannies, not all of whom were kind to him. One caregiver put him in a high chair inside a dark closet for hours when he was just a toddler.

When I was four, my status as the baby was updated to middle child with the birth of my other sister, Miranda. My parents were only twenty-four years old, with three young daughters to raise!

There is such an interesting dynamic that comes with being the middle child. There is real truth in the adage that we get lost in the shuffle.

Like most people, I do not recall much from my first four years. My memories begin around age five. (Oh, how I wish I could remember my first four years, to understand how they shaped me!)

One of my earliest memories is my first day of kindergarten. It was only a half day, and I remember being scared and uncertain, looking forward to noon, when I could go home. After we kids had settled in, the teacher asked me if I knew the ABCs. *Who doesn't know the ABCs?* I thought. I recited them confidently, already sure that I would be a good student.

A few hours passed, and it was time to go home. Parents began to arrive, and the classroom grew noisy with kids shouting and running into the arms of their moms and dads as though they hadn't seen each other in years. I waited. And waited. And waited. Eventually everyone left, including the teacher, and I was all alone, sitting on the steps outside my classroom. I remember being scared and crying quietly. *Where is everyone?* I thought. There was not even one teacher still around to help me.

Finally, after what felt like a century, my mom came. With a shrug she told me she'd forgotten that she had to pick me up. I'd been forgotten.

When I was about six years old, my family dynamic started to change. One night, I went outside to find my dad trying to drive his motorcycle up a tree. His eyes were wild, and he was saying strange and incomprehensible things. Frightened and confused, I ran inside to tell my mom. She did not seem surprised, which made me feel even more perplexed. She shooed me off and told me to not worry about it.

My dad's alcoholism and drug addiction ramped up. My father was not a happy drunk or functional alcoholic. When he was drinking, he became full-on psychotic—volatile, violent, and unpredictable. Even though he never laid a hand on me or called me names, I was always terrified, afraid he might hurt me or even kill me, never sure of what he might do. He'd be black-out drunk, acting crazy and totally unaware of what he was doing, and my older sister, Holly, was the only one who could calm him down. She had a way with him. She was a lot like him; she even looked like him. She would talk to him, hold his hand, stroke his hair, and settle him down. She could get him to a peaceful state. But she wasn't always there to protect us.

My mom was very rarely there to rescue us. Though I would call her at work and beg for her help, she never came.

The day after a blackout, my dad wouldn't remember anything. The previous night's craziness was never mentioned, like it never happened.

My family home was unstable and unsafe. My mom was not around most of the time, either out working or doing whatever it was she did to escape. Now, as an adult, I know that she was doing her best to survive. Still, in those moments, she abandoned me and my sisters.

When I was about seven, my dad took my younger sister, Miranda, and me out to dinner at a restaurant called Geno's. It was one of those hole-in-the-wall, dark Italian restaurants that always smelled of cigarette smoke. Miranda was only three years old at the time, a little redhead with bouncy curls who was always up for an adventure and still oblivious to the danger of our situation. My dad ordered one carafe of wine after another, and he quickly started getting loud and making a scene. Soon enough, the owner came over and asked us to leave. I looked around at the other diners, hoping that someone would step in. But no one stopped him; drunk as he was, they let him get into a car with a seven-year-old and three-year-old. He backed out of the parking spot with a jerk, swung the car around, and pulled out onto the road. As he sped down the street, I saw oncoming headlights as he swerved toward the guardrail. I started crying, certain that we were going to crash, that we were going to die. He slammed on the brakes.

"You don't like my driving?" he said. "Then why don't you drive?"

Now, on top of being scared, I was confused. Was he really going to make me drive? "No, that's OK," I told him, holding back my tears.

By the grace of God, we made it home. I didn't tell my mom. For a long time, I didn't tell anyone.

That was hardly the worst of it.

My sisters and I shared a loft bedroom upstairs and partitioned it off to give the illusion of having our own rooms. One time, while my mom was away in Mexico with one of her girlfriends, my dad had a "friend" over. She had a nice smile, plump rosy cheeks, and curly blonde hair. She seemed to really like my dad, and she was nice to me. She included me in the conversation, gave me hugs, and told me I was pretty. I really liked her. The next morning, I found her and my dad in my sister's bed (my sister was at a friend's house). I jumped on top of them, only to discover that they were naked. They laughed at my shock. I didn't truly understand what was happening, so I just stayed in bed with them.

My mom called that afternoon. I told her about Dad's new friend. I did not know something was wrong until I heard her reaction. She started crying and told me to go get my dad. In that moment, I knew I'd just revealed a secret. A secret that would unleash an infidelity war.

After that episode, my mom found a "friend" named Mitch. I believe he was in love with her. He helped my mom financially, and though I think she was fond of him, he was more her escape than anything. And she needed him. He would buy us gifts and take us places, and more importantly, he was kind.

One time he took me to the store. He put the car in neutral. "I'll be right back," he said, then got out and closed the door behind him. As soon as he walked away, the car started rolling backward, picking up speed. He ran back as fast as he could and pulled up the parking brake. I remember the look on his face, how concerned he'd been. I wasn't used to that. Then, one day, he was gone.

My parents tried bouts of separation. Often, we stayed with my dad at my dad's parents' house when my parents were trying to work things out. There I felt safer and more taken care of because they always had food around. One weekend, however, my grandparents were out of town. After my sisters and I went to bed, my dad left to go on a bender. In the morning, I woke up to find Janet, a longtime family friend and my grandparents' cleaning lady, standing outside the closed door of my grandparents' bedroom.

"Honey, don't go in there," she pleaded. I pushed past her and opened the door. My grandparents had separate single beds with their own televisions. My dad was passed out on my grandma's bed with an African American woman I had never seen before. Both were naked. I was so embarrassed.

What does Janet think? I wondered. In my limited experience, I had never seen an interracial relationship, and it added to my confusion and shock. Not only did I have to deal with the disappointment of the affair, but I had to process what all of that meant and what Janet thought.

My dad was a master manipulator and a liar. He would tell us that he was going to the store to get us Popsicles and just not come back. At every special occasion, especially holidays, we waited on pins and needles to see if he would get wasted. (He would.) After a bad binge, he would swear that he would stop drinking. Really, he would just make more of an effort to hide it for a little while. One time, my mom pulled down a ceiling tile and a ton of empty bottles fell on top of her.

The family tried interventions, and my dad went in and out of rehab over the next several years to try to get healthy and also salvage his marriage. Sometimes, I visited him there. It was always awkward and strained. I hated it. We would meet in these gathering rooms with fluorescent lights and long brown tables with cheap plastic chairs. It was dreary and empty. My dad would come out and sit across from me, and I never knew what to say. He always seemed somber and sad, like a lost dog waiting for someone to take him home.

When I was about eight years old, my dad picked me up from school, drove a few blocks away, pulled over on a neighborhood street, and put the car in park. He turned to me and said, "Your mom and I are getting divorced." I had little reaction. I was relieved, but more than that, I was numb. I knew the divorce was probably not going to make things better, that in all likelihood, it would make things worse.

My dad left that night, and then he was gone. Really gone. I did not care. In fact, I was glad that I didn't have to see him as much anymore. I rarely saw him, and when I did, I resisted. There were times I would not see him for months as he was still in and out of rehab centers. Over time, I started to build a wall of strength and control. I decided I was not going to take his behavior anymore. I would do things my way. I started focusing on school. At least I could control that.

After that, my sisters and I were left alone all the time, even more than we had been before. My mom was working and going to school for interior design and staying out of the house to escape her life. I was eight, Holly was ten, Miranda was four, and we were left to fend for ourselves. I once came home from school to find my little sister standing on top of the dining room table in only her underwear, dipping cubes of butter into a pile of sugar she had poured out all over the table.

Every day, we got ourselves to school in the morning. There was no one around to wake us up, make us breakfast, or give us a ride. We dressed ourselves (think dresses with pants underneath!) and walked to school. Our first meal of the day was the free school lunch available to low-income students. At night we cooked our own dinner, which was usually cereal or noodles with ketchup. If we were lucky, we had macaroni and cheese or hamburger meat with ketchup.

My mom worked as a cocktail waitress at night so she could go to school during the day. I admired that she wanted a career to better herself, but she didn't get home until two o'clock in the morning. Most nights, I waited up for her because I was afraid. We made friends with some workers at the nearby

Baskin-Robbins ice cream shop. They got off at eleven o'clock and would sometimes come by with ice cream. That gave me something to look forward to, as well as a sense of security, knowing that someone was checking in on us.

Almost immediately after my dad left, my mom's new boyfriend, Bob, moved in. Bob was tall with a thick mustache, shoulder-length brown hair and light eyes. He reminded me of Tom Selleck, circa *Magnum P.I.* in the eighties. They had probably been together for a while, but the day I met him was the day he moved in.

I did not like him from the start. He came in with the attitude of "this is my house now, you are going to follow my rules." But instead of my mom being around more since he was living with us, they would go out any chance they got. They started drinking and partying a lot, then they would come home and have LOUD sex. I would yell down from our loft bedroom, "Shut up!" while my mom moaned and wailed and screamed orgasmically all night. She didn't hear me, or she pretended not to. I felt invisible.

I asked my mom many times to have someone watch us while she was gone, because I got scared. Sometimes she did, sometimes she didn't. Many of the babysitters she found for us were neighbor kids who were not suitable for watching us. One girl took us to the park at midnight so she could meet up with boys, whom she brought back to our house to have sex with. Others were neighborhood boys. One babysitter in particular was about thirteen years old.

"Can I look in your vagina?" he asked one evening. "I want to know what I'll be fucking the first time I have sex."

"What?" I said, a bit unsure. "Um, no." He asked again, but my strength came through, and I stood my ground. "No!" I said, and this time I was sure. Thank goodness for my streak of defiance. After a while, I went up to my room, hoping that he wouldn't follow me. He didn't.

The next week, my mom announced that the same boy would be coming over to babysit.

"Please, Mom, don't let him come again," I said.

"Why not?"

"He . . . he . . . um . . . he asked me to show him my . . . you know."

My mom frowned. "Your what?"

"My . . . vagina." The last word was a whisper.

She paused, but not for long. "He probably meant no harm," she said. "And, anyway, no one else is available. So he'll have to do."

She left me on the steps leading up to my bedroom. I stayed there for hours, crying. Finally, I retreated to my room and did not come down. I did not want to see him, so I stayed alone up in my room until morning.

Over time, my fear and sense of helplessness turned to anger. Why was nobody helping me? Why could no one see me? One day, when I was around nine years old, I got called to the counselor's office at my elementary school.

"Leah," said the receptionist, "this nice lady here is from social services. She'd like to talk to you."

"OK," I said. She led me into a small office, where a woman was waiting. The woman sat behind the desk, and I sat down across from her. She started asking me questions about being neglected. Someone had called them and reported that we were not being cared for. She talked slowly and gently, trying to reassure me, tame any fear I might be having. But I was not scared.

Finally, someone saw it. Someone cared enough to say something. I knew exactly what social services was. I knew they could take me away from my family. Honestly, I did not care. I didn't hold back one bit. I told the lady all my woes, how I felt alone and how I did not like my mom's boyfriend and that we had no food. I wanted to be loved and seen so desperately. I wanted to feel safe and protected.

Afterward, social services called my house and made an appointment with my mom to come by and have a talk with the whole family. Of course, my mom cleaned the house from top to bottom. Remember, she was in school for interior design, so she was good at staging. She dressed us and herself up, making us look like the perfect family in clean clothes with our hair brushed, living in a spotless, beautifully decorated house. We were an attractive family, and it was easy to look the part. I was outraged, but my mom told us that we had better tell the social worker that everything was fine, or we would be taken away and separated forever. Fear got the better of me, and I went along with the charade.

The next day, my mom started trying to figure out who had called social services. She was convinced it was the neighbors up the street, whose house my little sister would play at from time to time. Years later I found out that it was one of my relatives. My own family! They said they knew social services would not take us away but wanted to put a good scare into my mom. Though I was shocked when I found out they'd called them, I was grateful. Someone whom I loved, loved me back.

Meanwhile, my mom's boyfriend, Bob, knew I did not like him. That was clear from the beginning. He would bully me and my sisters and tell us how ungrateful we were. It got worse after the social services incident. He started full-on verbally abusing us, calling us anything and everything, from snot-nosed brats to little bitches.

My mom seemed to enjoy this abuse. She wanted someone to take care of her too. She wanted to be seen too. She would tattle on us so that he would punish us. I remember the first time he hit me. I was up in my room, looking down the stairs. I had just gotten into a fight with my mom. I told her I hated her.

"Take it back," he said.

I shrugged.

"If you don't take it back, I will come and give you a reason to take it back," he said. I gave him a smirk. He ran up the stairs. I ran over to my sister's bed and lay down with my arms and legs up like a dead bug. He started hitting me and calling me a little bitch. I kicked him, trying to fend him off. Eventually he got tired and stumbled back down the stairs. I was sobbing.

"Mom!" I screamed. She came up and stood at the top of the stairs. She didn't say anything. "I'm going to run away!" She still didn't say anything, but she did step aside to make room for me to pass.

I ran away for about a half hour. No one came looking for me.

In fact, for most of my childhood, I felt unloved, unseen, and unprotected. Though my father and Bob were the ones who caused the drama, I constantly looked to my mother to protect me, and she neglected and abandoned me. I am sure she was trying to do her best. I believe people generally do their best with what they have and what they know. But her best left me feeling alone and scared.

There were some saving graces. I was headstrong, stubborn, defiant, and a natural leader, courageous and bold. There was a fire in me. That fire would carry me. Sometimes, when my mom was studying her designs, I would enter the room and she would look up from her drafting table with an annoyed smirk and try to shoo me away. Standing there, my feet firmly planted and my arms crossed, I would say, "I can stand here if I want to." Then, for as long as it took for me to feel like I'd made my point, I would not budge.

My aunts Yvonne and Maureen were also my saving graces, my inspiration. They were my dad's sisters. They were go-getters and seemed to have their lives together. My aunt Yvonne would take care of us when she could. She was in her early twenties and didn't have any kids. She was fun to be around. Together we would make yellow cake with chocolate frosting (still my favorite) and have sleepovers at my grandparents' house. She would give us back rubs, and we would talk and giggle. I loved being with her. My aunt Maureen was a lobbyist who lived in California. She didn't have kids of her own either, so she liked to spoil us. When she came to visit, she would buy us clothes and take us places. She was successful and fun. I wanted to be like her.

My dad's parents were also generous and loving. We called them Maka and Paka. Paka would light up when he saw me. He always called me Miss America and often took me and my sisters for ice cream. Maka showered us with gifts at Christmas and made our time together magical even in the midst of a crisis. Their love carried me through the hard times.

When I was around eleven, a new girl moved in next door. Jean was eighteen years old, with shiny black hair, light-blue eyes, and rosy cheeks. Her parents had just divorced, and she had decided to live with her dad.

One day she showed up at our door. "Hi!" she said. To me, she looked like an angel from heaven. "I'm new to the neighborhood. Come on over when you get a chance."

She didn't have to tell me twice. My sisters and I spent a lot of time there, just hanging out. To have an adult—or close to it—around was new to me, and something I had been craving for years. We baked cookies and watched TV, and sometimes she brought us dinner or helped us make something to eat. She was like a gift, a savior.

But she wrestled with her own demons too. I caught her purging every now and then and called her out on it. So I think we were there for her too. For me, she provided a source of stability for which I am forever grateful.

This first cycle, the Primal Cycle, sets the stage for our lives. Because my relationship with my mother was riddled with neglect and abandonment, and my father was so unwell, I did not feel seen or loved. Therefore, my path was directed and dictated by those tarnished relationships. The Primal Cycle would send me on a journey of many years to believe I was worthy of being seen. That's the thing—we learn our worth so early. If we do not feel worthy and do not have a foundation of security and love, we will spend years either repeating a cycle, caught in our false beliefs, or on a quest to unlearn them. Fortunately, I began my quest to unlearn my belief that I was unlovable, breaking the cycle of neglect and abandonment.

Primal Cycle Reflection Questions:

1. How was your mother's pregnancy? Were you wanted? Were you nurtured in the womb? Did you share the womb with a sibling?

2. How do you think the way you were formed affected how you feel seen, loved, and accepted?

3. During your childhood, who was your primary caretaker or caretakers? How were your relationships with them? What was the dynamic between your caretakers?

4. During your childhood, did you feel loved, safe, cared for, and protected? Did your primary caretaker make you feel seen?

5. What was your experience with the peripheral adults or caretakers in your life? Were you isolated, or could you depend on people outside your home?

The Struggle Cycle

"If there is no struggle, there is no progress."

—*Frederick Douglass*

The Struggle Cycle usually begins in adolescence. We are independent and self-sufficient enough to seek out external sources of love and attention from our parents and caregivers or, if they've proved unreliable, others. Just as most of us aren't prepared to pay our own bills and do our own grocery shopping at this stage, most of us aren't emotionally mature enough to find love and acceptance within ourselves. How we were seen—or not seen—by our caregivers during the Primal Cycle will dictate how much approval we seek externally and how we go about doing it.

The Struggle Cycle is all about trying to fit in and belong, figuring out who we are and if we are good enough, trying to find the happy ending. We tend to do the things people tell us to do, which includes our friends telling us *not* to do what our parents ask. We look everywhere but within ourselves to find acceptance and love. We think we're supposed to have it all figured out by early adulthood. So we navigate our lives and settle into societal and family pressures, and hope we are doing it right. This is why it is such a struggle.

Struggle Cycle survival can manifest in different ways. We might become extremely shy or clingy, or isolate ourselves, shut ourselves off from the world. We might become numb, using food, drugs, alcohol, sex, porn, television, or social media to escape reality or our feelings. We might become controlling or perfectionistic, which seem to be the most socially accepted survival techniques.

My survival mode was control. I was all about perfectionism and overachieving. If I could control my life, be the best and succeed in all facets of my life, then maybe someone would see me, someone would love me fully like I needed to be loved. Better yet, maybe my mom and dad would see me.

Starting in elementary school, I got straight As, took on leadership roles like Associated Student Body president and patrol crossing-guard captain (that was a big deal), and was a social activist. When I found out that the flag football team didn't allow girls, I lobbied hard and finally won the case.

I was the ringleader of my friend group. I remember buying a teal checkered fleece pullover, the absolute height of tween fashion. So my best friends, Kate and Melissa, wanted to get teal fleece pullovers too. Then all of our other friends wanted them. As the ringleader, it was up to me to approve who could be in the jacket club.

I'm the first to admit that my leadership skills were a little rough around the edges. But trial and error is how kids figure out life during the Struggle Cycle. At the time, I was looking more for attention, control, and to be seen, rather than to truly lead.

Around this time I began to get boy crazy. In fifth grade I started playing spin the bottle and making out with boys in the closet. Despite my popularity, I had a poor body image. I was a chubby kid, and boys (and my older sister) teased me about it. It was one of the things that I could not yet control.

I thought that if I could be perfect, my mom would see me. But the more I strove to achieve, the more invisible I became. Meanwhile, Holly was getting Ds in school, and Miranda was stealing and smoking cigarettes. She was eight. My mom focused all of her attention on them, putting me on the back burner because I wasn't causing trouble. My parents thought I had it all figured out, that I didn't need them, when really my efforts amounted to me waving my arms and screaming, *Look over here! Can you see me? See me! See me!* But instead of being seen, I became even more invisible.

In fifth grade, I entered my first beauty pageant, Miss Washington National Pre-Teen. That was the first of three pageants that I entered. What better way to be seen than to put myself on display?

I did jazz dancing for the talent portion of the competition. For the evening gown ceremony, all the other girls wore tiaras. I wore a big blue derby hat. I wanted to stand out. My uncle walked with me during the ceremony, since my dad was in rehab or off the grid somewhere. I won third place out of hundreds of girls.

My mom left early, I am not sure why. But she passed me off to my uncle. I felt disappointed but not surprised. My uncle drove me home that night. I could see him nodding off, then waking up with a jerk of his head. My big trophy sat next to me in the back seat, but instead of feeling proud, I felt empty and alone. There was no trophy big enough to give me a sense of safety and security. I did not know how to create that for myself yet.

At the end of sixth grade, my mom told us we would be moving from Spokane to Kirkland for Bob's new job. I was devastated. Would people like me there? Would they call me fat? Would I be popular? What about my dad, my friends, my neighbor Jean, and the rest of my family? Would I see them again?

Though junior high was still the emotional nightmare for me that it is for most people, I actually assimilated quite easily. Within a few weeks of starting school, I made a whole new crew of friends and had a seat at the popular kids' table. I kept up my straight As and signed up for the student body cabinet; I eventually ran for student body president and won. I fell into that role seamlessly.

I prided myself on how many friends said hi or hugged me in the halls. I would literally keep count. Obviously, this was an attempt to measure love, a way to get validation.

At school, I got lots of attention. I relied on those external sources to fuel me.

At home, it was a different story. My mom and Bob were drinking and fighting a lot, and mostly I just did my best to stay out of their way. My mom started drinking a bottle of wine every night. Unlike my dad, she was a functional alcoholic. I reasoned that it wasn't so bad because she was able to work and didn't go crazy on us. But she'd often get drunk and cry and say things like, "Why do you hate me? You should hate your dad! He was the one who hurt this family!"

She blamed him for all our family dysfunction. She never saw her own part in it, never owned her behavior or apologized or recognized her abandonment of us, her selfishness. She felt she did the best she could. She probably did. Maybe what she gave was all she could give during those hard years of my father's alcoholism. But she never recognized that it might not have been what we needed.

Bob started getting more aggressive as we got older. When my mom got drunk and weepy, instead of being sympathetic, I got annoyed and angry with her, and then Bob would step in and verbally abuse me for not being "nice" to my mother. One time, he asked me to apologize to her. I refused. So he took me by the neck, threw me up against the door, and called me a fucking cunt. I was thirteen years old.

Even after witnessing that kind of behavior, my mom wanted us to love Bob. She would say things like, "He has been more of a father to you than your own dad" and "He loves you like his own." I didn't believe her. Where was the evidence of this thing she called love?

It was true that Bob was around more than my dad. My dad had bouts of sobriety, during which I saw him more often. He had been doing well for a while when my mom told me, one morning before school in seventh grade, that my dad had relapsed and flatlined the night before. The medics had brought him back from beyond with a shock from a defibrillator.

I went to school in a daze. All through my first-period language arts class, I kept thinking about how my dad had died the night before. He was told that if he ever drank again, he would die for certain. The ambiguity and uncertainty were torture. Would he leave me? Would my dad abandon me forever? Fortunately, he never drank again.

As things got worse at home, I threw myself more and more into school, extracurricular activities, and hanging out with my friends. I had tons of friends but never felt fully connected to any of them. I had a couple of close friends, Kelsey and Belinda, but they'd made it clear that they were already best friends and that I was their second-best friend. I did not have a best friend, someone who looked at me as their number one and about whom I felt the same. I was trying so hard to find that external source to love me, fill me up, see me.

I started experimenting with drugs and alcohol that year, in seventh grade. For a long time, I stayed away from alcohol—my mom and dad were great examples of why *not* to drink. So I smoked pot instead. Not because it numbed me or made me feel all that great, but to fit in. I didn't want to be some goody-two-shoes wallflower. That was ultimately why I started drinking alcohol too. It was fun for the first few hours, when I got a good buzz on. But once I went from buzzed to wasted, there was always drama, someone holding my hair back as I puked on the bathroom floor, some bad behavior I'd regret the next day. I would wake up the next morning depressed and hungover and worried sick about what others thought of me. Had I done anything stupid? I hated it and never understood why people thought it was cool, but I kept doing it to fit in.

I also met a boy. His name was Connor. He wasn't totally into me at first. I chased him, but he liked my friend Kelsey. Kelsey was blonde with blue eyes, and she had a "perfect" body.

One day she and I were swimming at the community pool when Connor showed up. Later that night, after changing out of my bikini and into some comfy sweats, I talked to him on the phone. "What do think of my body?" I eventually worked up the nerve to ask.

"Top half is good, bottom half needs work," he said.

So I stopped eating. I starved myself during school hours, then ate when I got home. I was certain that Connor would like me if I lost weight. So little in my life was under my control, but along with my grades, I could control that. *Be more perfect,* I thought, *and then someone will love me.*

It worked. Connor started liking me. He was a wrestler, and he would run to my house wearing a black garbage bag under his clothes so that he'd sweat in order to make weight. He would show up at my door drenched and out of breath and eager to see me. He was playful with me, tender and sweet.

Connor was first person with whom I felt I was their first priority. With him I was not a middle child or a second-best friend—I was number one. It was the closest thing to real love that I had ever experienced.

But my bliss was interrupted in eighth grade, when my friend Kelsey was sent away to boarding school. Her parents thought she was getting out of control and just shipped her off without letting her say goodbye. It was the first time I felt loss and grief of such great magnitude. I felt like she had died, like she had been ripped out of my life, like she'd abandoned me. My heart was torn.

After Kelsey left, I became good friends with Andrea. She was the closest thing I had to a best friend for many years. She had another best friend, but she was mine. She was one of those girls who was ahead of her time. She was striking, with hair that was two-toned—platinum blonde on top and dark brown in the back. She got noticed. She dated older guys. She started having sex when she was thirteen, with sixteen- and seventeen-year-olds. She learned how to drive and started sneaking out in her brother's old brown Toyota Corolla at fourteen. She was the person people came to for advice. She seemed to know all the answers.

I had many first experiences with Andrea. During the summer we went up to Birch Bay, in Washington near the Canadian border, where her family had a cabin. We would stand outside the convenience store and ask men going inside to buy beer or California Coolers for us, then get drunk and chase boys. Everything was about getting male attention. I thought somehow a boy would come rescue me, save me, complete me.

Most of my friends started having sex in junior high. I did not. Even though Connor and I had gotten serious and I loved him, I refrained from having sex. It was not a decision based on religious scruples or some kind of moral judgment. It was just a matter of me being afraid. What if I gave myself to someone, and then he decided that I wasn't good enough, or that he didn't really love me? What if he left me? I could not bear the thought of being left again.

Though that year was full of growing pains, at the same time I had such a feeling of freedom, of burgeoning independence. I was in that stage of breakaway, when kids come to know that one day in the future they will no longer have to conform to their parents' wishes. I realized that one day I would be on my own and able to make my own decisions. That someday I could be myself.

As we headed into high school for tenth grade, Connor and I were still dating on and off. To my surprise, we were voted homecoming prince and princess. I started dreaming of the homecoming parade, of driving in a convertible with the top down on a perfect night, sitting in the back waving and smiling, everyone lined up along the road to watch. I always put such high expectations on moments like that.

That night, Connor showed up as planned, and I was annoyed rather than elated. I didn't want to be with him. He didn't do anything wrong; I was just consumed by my own expectations.

It was pouring. In the back of the "fancy" Peugeot that was donated for the parade, we stuck our heads out the sunroof. The rain soaked my fancy hairdo, smeared my makeup, and drenched the top of my dress. Far fewer people showed up than had in my imagination. All in all, it was nothing like what I thought it would be. I'd been highly attached to my anticipated outcome, so I was really disappointed.

After that, Connor and I finally parted ways. He started dating someone else but tried to convince me to wait for him.

He strung me along for a while, but I eventually let go. I started chasing boys who did not like me back. I had my heart broken again and again. Why would no one love me?

At the end of my sophomore year, I tried out for the varsity cheerleading squad, and I made it! I achieved one of my ultimate goals. I was stoked.

That summer, going into my junior year, I met a boy named Eddie. We met at a local hangout, Pietro's Pizza. It was one of those love-at-first-sight moments, when everything slows down and you can't see anything but each other. I remember him walking toward me and everything else around us fading out. There was only him.

Eddie was perfect. He was cute, he was on the football team, and he drove a Jeep. But more than that, he had the family of my dreams. His mom stayed home to take care of him and his younger brother and sister, and his dad was an accountant. Finally, the perfect boy and the perfect family, and they all seemed to love me just as much as I loved them.

Eddie and I got serious right away. We spent as much time together as possible that summer, and when school started up again, we hung out every afternoon that I didn't have cheerleading and he didn't have football practice. We would hang out in his room on his bed and dream of our life together. Within a few months, we had picked out the names of our kids. He even gave me a promise ring!

But we weren't so romantic at school. Eddie basically ignored me. He didn't want to be seen with me, let alone engage in public displays of affection. I wasn't allowed to kiss him or sit with him in the commons, and he never showed up for my cheerleading performances. I was confused.

After school, I was his everything, but during school hours I was nothing. Of course, I thought it was my fault, that I was doing something wrong. It took me many years to figure out that it was about Eddie's ego, not some sort of flaw within me.

He cared so much about what other people thought. He was afraid of being called "pussy-whipped," and he was desperate to maintain the image of a stud who was not attached or bound to anyone.

In his family—and society at large at the time—in all relationships, the woman was supposed to be behind the man. But I was a strong woman, a high achiever and independent. He couldn't reconcile who I was with who he thought I should be, or who he was with who he thought he should be. His pride caused us both to suffer.

I didn't have any inkling of this at the time, so I chased him instead of letting go of the relationship. I put up with it because he always came back to me when we were behind closed doors. And because I loved being at his house with his family. They had real family dinners, with everyone saying grace beforehand, and talking, and eating a meal that his mom had prepared. I reveled in this manifestation of my ideal family.

There were times when Eddie role-played as my dad. He would hold me and put my head in his lap. "You're my baby girl," he would say.

"Daddy, do you love me?" I would say.

He would respond, "I love you."

"Daddy, will you ever leave me?" I would ask.

He would say, "I will never leave you."

He was the first person who vowed not to leave me, but still—and for good reason—I was constantly afraid of him leaving me. So much so that my mom called my dad and made him talk to me. In the call, my dad apologized for all that he had put me and my sisters through. He couldn't remember most of what he had done, but he recognized the harm he'd caused and that he had made me fearful of loss and abandonment. He saved our relationship that day. By him owning his part in the challenges of my life, I felt seen and more capable of forgiveness.

The deal was sealed with Eddie when we took our relationship to the next level. I gave myself to someone in the most intimate way I knew how. I was in it for life. I was seventeen years old.

Not that sex changed anything as far as our distance during school hours went. We did not appear to be together, but behind closed doors, we were fully committed.

High school wasn't all about boyfriend drama, though. I had two jobs in high school. My first job was at a tanning salon; later on, I worked as a hostess at a Mexican restaurant. I had tons of friends to hang out with who carted me around to social activities. Much of my time was spent at sporting events or cheerleading practice. The other cheerleaders were my posse, and the sport gave me purpose. I began to see how leading and inspiring were part of me and made me happy.

I could drive, but I did not have my own car until my senior year, when my dad bought me a green Ford Pinto. I was embarrassed—it did not fit the image I was trying to convey—and didn't see the generosity of his gift. As luck would have it, the car ran for only a few weeks.

As I grew in my independence, I moved further away from my mom and Bob, who were now married, and into my own life. Holly had become an alcoholic and Miranda struggled with cocaine and marijuana abuse. My mom was busy dealing with them and becoming more enmeshed in codependency. None of them were looking within themselves to deal with their own wounds. It was easier for me to avoid them and look for external validation elsewhere.

I graduated high school with a 3.98 GPA. (I cried hysterically when I got my one and only B in geometry.) I had near-perfect grades, the ideal boyfriend, lots of friends, and cheerleader status. But it wasn't enough—even with all that, I still didn't feel seen.

One night I went with my mom to her work party. There was a woman named Celeste there who read palms.

"Can I read your palm, sweetie?" she asked. I hesitantly gave her my hand. She studied my palm for a few moments. When she looked up, she had big tears running down her face. I was scared. What did she see?

She looked me square in the eye. "You are going to help a lot of people," she said. "And you will do great things in the world."

Her words stayed with me. But more than that, she saw me. Really saw me, to the depth of my soul. She believed I was meant for greatness, so I believed it too. Her words helped shape my life and gave me the inspiration to stay open to possibilities and seek my purpose. I never saw her again.

The summer after graduation was an uncertain time for Eddie and me. He was going to go to community college and I was going to go to the University of Washington. I could feel his insecurity about our going to different schools. One day, in his room, we sat on the floor and bawled, afraid of the looming changes. Would we be able to maintain our relationship? Would we meet other people? I had not received any scholarships and would be living at home. In my heart, I wanted to live on campus, but I rationalized that this was better because I would be closer to Eddie.

As soon as college started, I felt disconnected from my old life. I was at a huge university, taking weeder classes (classes that weed out the weaker students). All my old friends were now scattered around the country. I was commuting back and forth, working at the same Mexican restaurant, and studying all the time.

Just when I could've used him the most, Eddie went MIA. I didn't hear from him for weeks. I knew he was avoiding my calls, but there was nothing I could do. As he drifted further away from me, a coworker named Paul started giving me all kinds of attention. He was a huge flirt, and I just soaked it up. We began to spend more time together, and I rationalized that we were just friends so it was no big deal. But I was definitely attracted to him. One night after work, we took a walk and he kissed me on a bridge in the park in the moonlight. I felt weak in the knees.

After that, I really considered leaving Eddie, but I felt like he deserved another chance because we had been together so long and I was committed to him. Ultimately, I was afraid to lose him, too, *and* I did not want to be the abandoner. I gave him an ultimatum: either he would stay connected or I would let him go. He bucked up and vowed to be more attentive. The relationship with Paul went no further.

I flailed through the first two years of college, looking for a way to belong. I made one close friend, Dana. She was in the Greek system, but she wasn't the typical sorority girl. She avoided affiliated events and made her own friends outside her house. We spent a ton of time together. One of my best times in college was a road trip I took with her to her home in Encinitas, California, for spring break. Ultimately, though, with her I enacted some of my codependent tendencies: I got clingy and held tight but then grew weary and started to pull away, at which point she felt slighted. My not calling her on her birthday was the last straw and the end of our friendship.

In my second year of college, Eddie and I moved in together, into a small apartment with another couple. Though the guy was one of Eddie's best friends, the situation wasn't ideal. Eddie's friend gave me the creeps. He would sprawl on the sofa watching television for hours wearing shorts that were so short I could see his testicles. His girlfriend was also a control freak, so we clashed. And they had a cat. Eddie did not like it, and I was allergic. We lasted a few months there, then got our own place.

Eddie and I quickly fell into a routine. It was clear we were more like roommates than partners, that we were just going through the motions. We didn't talk much or even fight. We rarely had sex. But it was safe, and I knew no other way. Still, I felt trapped. Everyone thought we would get married, that we were the perfect couple. We fit the image, and I wanted to uphold it. I was doing what I thought I was supposed to do. However, I was complacent and lonely.

My friend Andrea from high school was a saving grace. We hung out a lot, sitting around drinking coffee at Denny's or eating rice and beans at the local Azteca. I'd begun to obsess about my junior high boyfriend, Connor. I thought I was still in love with him, and Andrea and I endlessly talked about how I could find ways to see him or work up the guts to call him. She listened to me hash out all my angst and loneliness.

Eventually, the talk became action. I would call Connor and hang up. I would seek him out at parties. I would listen to music and cry about him. He was my long-lost love, the love I couldn't have. Back then, I didn't realize he was just my *representation* of love. I took his role in my imagination literally. He was something tangible and real that I could latch on to. Since I was not feeling loved by Eddie, I sank my hooks into the idea of Connor.

I craved the attention that my boyfriend wasn't giving me. I started going out with my old high school friends a lot. I would flirt, dance dirty, and occasionally kiss other guys while we were out. My friends judged me for my behavior since I was in a relationship. At the time, I could not make sense of why I was doing what I was doing. I did not understand my own loneliness. I thought it was just part of who I was. I didn't realize I was trying to be seen, loved, noticed.

To deal with that internal dissonance, I compartmentalized my life. With my friends I was a certain way, and with Eddie I was another way. He never came out with me, instead preferring to stay home by himself, his own loneliness and low self-esteem keeping him from being seen. In fact, some of my college friends did not believe that Eddie actually existed. They teased me and said I made him up. In four years of college, they never met him.

Junior year, I applied and got in to the Michael G. Foster School of Business at UW. It was a highly competitive school, ranked top ten in the nation. My classes shrank from a huge ocean to a small fishbowl. I decided to major in accounting. It wasn't that I loved accounting. I actually failed my first accounting midterm and struggled with the first few classes. But it was the most competitive major. There were only a few jobs for accounting graduates, and I wanted one of them. Maybe I would fit in somewhere; maybe I would be truly seen in that job, at least by my peers.

I got involved quickly. I ran for vice president of the accounting fraternity, Beta Alpha Psi. I didn't know a lot of people, but I ran anyway. And I won. Being in that leadership role got me noticed. I made more friends, went to more social events, and best of all, started being courted by companies who wanted me to work for them. I felt I had purpose and a sense of belonging.

My new friends, Mandy and Sara, and I spent hours studying for the Certified Public Accountant (CPA) tests and eating chocolate chip cookies. Those women were smart, the ones who set the curve and whom everyone wanted to hire. I always felt a little out of my league with them, as well as playing second fiddle. That was sort of my jam: being the third wheel, the odd man out, the one on the back burner. They did their best to make me feel included, but they were in sororities and I lived with Eddie on the Eastside. Even so, they were—and still are—dear friends to me.

The three of us went through college recruiting together. College recruiting was the process we went through to be placed for our jobs/careers after we graduated. It was cutthroat, with only twenty-seven public accounting jobs up for grabs. It involved a lot of mingling, going to events, networking, and interviewing. Mandy and Sara landed jobs at Big Six accounting firms. I got a job at a local regional firm called Clark Nuber. It was not my top choice, but I was really excited to get a job in public accounting. I felt like I had made it. I'd gotten a good education and a good job, so I was going to be happy now, right?

Struggle Cycle Reflection Questions:

1. What's your survival mode? Are you shy or clingy? Do you numb your feelings? Do you control?
2. How has that survival mode affected your relationships?
3. What external sources have you continually sought out to feel belonging, love, and acceptance? Were there behaviors you repeated over and over in an attempt to be seen?
4. How much do you try to fit in or keep up with your peers? Is there an image of yourself you're trying to convey?
5. When did you start breaking away from your parents? When did you realize that someday your life would be your own?
6. What representations of love did you view as real?
7. What did you think would make you happy?
8. Was there anyone who really saw you during the Struggle Cycle?

Conform Cycle

"The highest forms of love are inevitably totally free choices and not acts of conformity."

—*M. Scott Peck,* The Road Less Traveled: A New Psychology of Love, Traditional Values and Spiritual Growth

In the Conform Cycle, we see things the way we want to see them, not as they are. We are still looking for external validation, putting up masks and facades, and not looking within.

Unfortunately, this is the place most of us stay. We get stuck here because we invest so much time, money, and effort into repeating societal and familial norms and values. Enacting those norms and values is more likely to bring us all the things we're supposed to want. So why would we do otherwise? Most of us live the lives expected of us until the day we die. It takes great courage to break free, to shed the standards thrust upon us by the culture at large, our parents, our parents' parents, and so on down the line.

———

Right as college was ending, Eddie came home and told me we had to look at a new opportunity. He'd been approached by someone who told him he could be financially independent. My first words were, "Is it Amway?"

I knew of Amway, a multilevel marketing business, through that same uncle who had walked with me in the pageants. He and his wife had been in it for a long time and were doing quite well. I knew that the company had a reputation for being a pyramid scheme, but my aunt and uncle seemed to be successful. So although I was not totally into it, I agreed to explore the opportunity. I wanted so much for Eddie to step up and show me that he was a part of our relationship in the way I thought he should be, as the leader of the family, just like his dad.

We got drawn into the business almost instantly, quickly conforming to their standards. We stopped watching television, and we went to meetings and rallies all the time. We fully drank the Amway Kool-Aid.

I was working sixty to seventy hours a week in my new career at the accounting firm, and I knew that wouldn't be sustainable forever. Amway was heavily based in the Christian faith and encouraged women to stay home and men to take care of their families. I bought into that and began to dream of being a stay-at-home mom. Both of us were seeking to settle into a conformity that was familiar. We wanted security, and that was what Amway promised.

I knew, too, that there were some standard next steps in life after college. It was time to do what I thought all people do: get married and have babies. It was time to settle down.

Eddie and I got married on June 14, 1997, in the Catholic Church. That was what his parents wanted. I was not Catholic. Though both my parents grew up Catholic, they'd turned to a nondenominational Christian faith and I was raised that way. Eddie and I were twenty-three.

It was a big traditional wedding; the guests were mostly high school friends and some of our new Amway friends, plus a bunch of our parents' friends whom I didn't know. I wore a fancy white wedding dress embossed with beads and sequins, a veil, and a ten-foot train.

My mom insisted that Bob walk me down the aisle. "Bob is going to walk you down the aisle, right?" she inquired.

"I want my dad to walk me down the aisle."

"You should have both of them, one on each arm."

"I don't want that, Mom," I said. "I want just one person walking me down the aisle."

"Bob will be crushed. He loves you. He is your father," she said, laying on the guilt.

"No, he's not, Mom. My father is alive and well, and I want him."

"But . . . but . . . Bob just has to."

I finally agreed to let Bob walk me partway down the aisle, then be intercepted by my dad, who gave me away.

Conformity is abiding by all the rules even when they are not what we really want. Ultimately, I resented the decision. As I walked down the aisle, I couldn't wait for the interception to take place. Walking with my dad was my heart's true desire.

After, we took a Caribbean cruise for our honeymoon. Instead of being romantic, it was mostly awkward and strained. Eddie spent a bunch of time playing blackjack at the casino while I stayed in the room. We were young, naive, and immature.

A year later, we bought our first house with the help of Eddie's parents. We got a couple of dogs. I was busy building my career, and Eddie was working as a landscaper with my stepdad, Bob, and trying to make something out of the Amway business. We thought we were doing what we were supposed to be doing. We kept the Amway business going for several years, but nothing came of it, and I started to get antsy and did not want to waste any more time or money. So we stopped.

I also started getting tired of the demands of public accounting. I had tried to get my CPA license three times and failed the exam each time. So I decided to leave my job at Clark Nuber. I landed a new job in private industry as the assistant controller for a residential homebuilder. They gave me the title and the pay, but my responsibilities were mostly grunt work. I wasn't using any of the skills I had learned in public accounting, and I quickly started to get depressed. I felt stuck.

I turned to fitness for some relief. I met Dawni Rae at a kickboxing class. She was an amazing instructor and an inspiration. She was a spitfire, tiny but crazy strong, with curly black hair and a giant smile. I started following her to all her classes and asked her to be my trainer. After that, we became really good friends—and best friends years later.

Getting in shape gave me more confidence. It helped me realize how unhappy I was and that I needed to keep learning and growing or I would continue to feel stagnant and depressed. Movement does that. It gets us unstuck from our fears and a scarcity mindset, and into an expanse of love and openness in our lives. I decided to go back to my old job at Clark Nuber, but in the tax department instead of the audit department, where I'd been before. I made a commitment to pass my CPA exam and put all my effort back into that career. I had so many growth opportunities there. I could eventually make my way to partner. I could make a ton of money and work myself up the ranks. I was sick of sitting on the sidelines. It was time for me to make shit happen.

Shortly after returning to Clark Nuber, I passed the CPA exam and made plans to get on the partner track. I also created a college recruiting program for our firm. I wanted our firm to be a presence on college campuses and recruit the most talented students. I felt empowered by taking the reins on that project, and I could see how I was able to inspire people to be their best while I was also building community. I met with some resistance because it took me away from billable hours, but ultimately the firm appreciated the groundwork I laid for bringing in quality employees.

By this time, I had accepted that I was going to be the breadwinner in our family. Eddie had broken away from my stepdad's landscaping business and created his own because their relationship had become strained (hence the sage advice to not work with your family). Many of his clients came from my referrals. So there I was, making the money, paying the bills, bringing in my husband's clients, and doing most of the household work too. (Eddie cooked, thank goodness.)

As usual, I was doing too much, overfunctioning, as a way to maintain control. I had given Eddie the chance to step up when we'd been involved in Amway. But when he didn't, I was done. It was time for me to run the show. I believed that holding our lives together was all on me. My overfunctioning revved up to superspeed. That did not do much to improve Eddie's self-esteem or initiative. He would get depressed and I would do more. He could go for days not talking to me, just hiding away in his shed in the backyard or in any other room of the house that I was not in.

My love language is physical touch, but the more I controlled him (and every aspect of my life), the more Eddie pulled away from me. We scheduled sex for once a week, and it was the same each time. Anytime I went to hug him, he would push me away.

To me, that felt like punishment. Was he punishing me, or was he punishing himself? Likely both. He resented me and I resented him. We did not realize the jam we were in, the disservice we were both doing to ourselves and our marriage.

I felt trapped and lonely but was terrified of losing what we'd built. So I just stayed. Stuck.

After about seven years of marriage, I went to Las Vegas for a bachelorette party and met a man named Marc from Orange County, California. He was wild and handsome and seemed to think that I was amazing too. We were both married, but we flirted right to the edge of inappropriate. For the record, we never crossed the line. But when I got home, we started to email each other every day. We would make plans to try to see each other. We were both lonely. This fantasy consumed me.

I brought up the situation to Andrea, and she tried to convince me to separate from Eddie. She'd been hearing about my woes for years, and she said that it was time to leave. I listened to her advice and started to make plans to separate. Then my period was late.

I had never had regular periods, but the time between them was longer than usual. Eddie and I had not been using protection for about two years. We wanted to have a baby, or rather, we thought we should want to have a baby. We didn't exactly try, but we didn't not try either.

Right before the wedding of the bachelorette from the party in Vegas, I took a pregnancy test. It was positive. I cried; I was sitting there alone on the toilet sobbing, not because I was happy but because I was scared. I knew now that I would have to stay.

Like I did for any of my projects, once I decided I was in, I was in, and I turned my entire focus to my pregnancy. The first trimester I suffered from morning sickness and gained a bunch of weight. I didn't love being pregnant like some women do, but I loved the little one growing inside of me.

Marc visited me when I was about four months along. We met up at a restaurant, and afterward he tried to kiss me in the car. I flipped out and left immediately.

Eddie and I did not find out the sex of the baby—we wanted it to be a surprise. On March 12, 2002, I woke up early thinking I had peed my pajamas. Eddie had already gone to work. I was still almost a month away from my due date. I went to the bathroom and each time I tried to get up from the toilet, I felt more "pee" come out.

I called my mom and she told me that she thought my water had broken. My mom had just gotten home from helping deliver my younger sister Miranda's twin boys the night before. Miranda and I had had the same due date. There was something cosmic about us both going into labor early and at almost the same time.

I was not at all prepared. I called the hospital and they told me to take my time. "Don't panic," they said. I tried to get ahold of Eddie but couldn't. I eventually got through, and he hurried home and whisked me off to the hospital. I was a few days away from a major tax deadline, and ever conscientious, I called in to work to arrange my affairs.

My mom wanted to be in the room for the birth. I did not want her in there, but once again I caved to family pressure. She wanted Bob in the room, too, but I stood my ground on that one. I could not fathom him seeing me in that way. Eddie, Andrea, Holly, and my mom were the people I allowed in the room. My mom tried to nurture me by putting ChapStick on my lips, but I batted her hand away in annoyance. Andrea and Holly were my cheerleaders while I took a hot bath and had an epidural. Eddie stepped in to support me when I pushed for an hour. After six hours at the hospital, Alexis Kennedy Zaccaria was born. She was small at five pounds, six ounces, but she was healthy. I'd never felt love like the kind I felt in those first moments of her life. She was a miracle. I will never forget the feeling of holding her in my arms and touching her skin to mine. I wept with the deepest sense of gratitude all the way to my core. This little human who had grown inside me: she would be my most precious gift.

The days that followed were amazing. Even with an infant to take care of, maternity leave felt very luxurious to me. Yes, I was not sleeping much, but the days I spent just staring at her, rocking her, and walking around with her seemed so spacious. Time slowed down. She was an awesome baby. She slept well, ate well, and was always happy. She's pretty much been that way ever since.

After three months, I went back to work. I decided to go back part time. Part time in public accounting means only forty to forty-five hours a week. I was able to work one day at home. I had always held it all together, and I would do the same now.

My good friend and neighbor was a stay-at-home mom with three little girls. She cared for Alexis while I worked. Leaving my daughter that first day was surreal. Alexis cried at the top of her lungs as I walked away. Eddie got off work at around two o'clock, so I took solace in the fact that she would not be away from us all day. He loved Alexis and took good care of her, and he was able to spend a lot of time with her since he wasn't working the same long hours I was. He was, and continues to be, an active father to her.

The next five years were a juggling act. I was a CPA, mother, wife, and friend. In each of those roles, I showed up differently. But in each of them, I overfunctioned as usual. I was consumed with looking the part and doing it best. Of course, when it's all about appearances, the insides of our experiences get to be hollow and lonely. I was everything and nothing at all.

In my CPA role, I was strong and intimidating, a go-getter always climbing toward the top. The people I managed were a little afraid of me. I admit, my expectations were really high. I had the best clients and got promoted early. I stayed late and worked weekends.

In my wife role, I was head of the household. I took charge. I scheduled all activities, planned everything, and took care of everyone. I was rigid and hard. Sometimes, Eddie would say, "Get the stick out of your ass." My constitution is fiery, and if I'm out of balance, I come off as angry and stressed. I was constantly out of balance at home. I did all the tasks that traditional wives are supposed to do and more, but not with a smile on my face.

In my friend role, I was funny and wild. I would go out and cut loose, flirt, drink, and dance. I was a good listener and fun to be around. Being a friend was my way to escape.

In my mother role, I was Suzy Homemaker. The house always had to be perfect. I took Alexis on playdates and to parks and bought her anything she wanted. I did the Christmas shopping before Thanksgiving and had all the presents wrapped and under our two Christmas trees—one upstairs, one downstairs—before we finished the leftover turkey and stuffing.

The relationship between my stepdad and Eddie was still strained, stemming from when they worked together. Eddie was too afraid to confront him, so I had to hear about it for weeks before a family gathering, then Eddie would put on a happy face and pretend everything was fine. It was a huge burden for me. Even though it wasn't mine to carry, I carried it anyway.

More than anything, I was in love with the *idea* of family. I reveled in traditions and looking the part. But whenever I was with my mother and stepfather, all my hard work fell apart. Every holiday turned into a drinking fest and an emotional hijacking. My mom would drink too much wine and then start in with the psychological warfare. She was infamous for saying, "I do everything for you girls, and you don't love me." True to form, she would blame our family woes on my dad and never take ownership of her part in the dysfunction. My sisters and I would roll our eyes or get angry, and my stepdad would jump in and tell us what ungrateful bitches we were. Year after year, I would decorate the house, envisioning the perfect holiday: everyone contently drinking eggnog in front of a roaring fire, all in matching sweaters, singing Christmas carols. Instead, it would always end with my mom drunkenly weeping and my stepdad red in the face. My sisters had bouts of sobriety, but they were on-again, off-again. Rest assured that if my sisters were also drunk, everything was much worse.

It had been the exact same thing when I was a kid at extended-family gatherings on my mom's side. Everyone got wasted and ended up crying or fighting. It was a learned pattern for my mom, and it continued into our nuclear family. For whatever reason, we always came back for more. We knew no other way.

I took solace in Eddie's family for many years. But no family is perfect, especially the ones we put on a pedestal. Often those are the ones that are the most dysfunctional, but either we can't see it or they're better at hiding it. A few years into our marriage, one night we heard someone crawling across the roof and then knocking on the window to our family room upstairs. Startled, we went to the window and saw that it was Eddie's sister. We pulled her inside. She was wild-eyed and manic, holding a bag of candy bars and talking incoherently. We calmed her down and called their parents.

She was admitted to the hospital and diagnosed with a mental illness. Later, she claimed she was abused by her other brother (not Eddie). That claim devastated the family; Eddie and his parents were shocked by his sister's accusations. She blamed her mental illness on him, and the whole thing tore their family apart. The other brother was cast out, and no one ever talked about it. At family gatherings, the elephant in the room took the form of the empty dining room chair where their brother and son used to sit. Eddie's mom's blood pressure skyrocketed, and she worried all the time. Yet no one would get help. They just kept going to church and putting on a facade of the perfect family. Eddie's sister ruled the roost, and everyone walked on eggshells to appease her. The family that I had once admired and been so grateful to be a part of had diminished. I caught a glimpse through their perfect veneer to the trouble and tragedy within.

Conform Cycle Reflection Questions:

1. What societal and familial norms do you conform to? Do they truly feel like they align with your deepest desires? If not, where do your desires differ from those norms?
2. What things did you see as you wanted to see them? Were they embedded in you? Were they true?
3. What roads or paths did you take because you felt like you should or had to?
4. When you felt stuck, did you remain passive due to the pressures of this conformity? If not, what kinds of actions did you take? Were they helpful?
5. Do you worry what others will think if you change?
6. Was there a moment when you almost allowed yourself to want what you truly wanted or to see things as they truly were? Did you turn a blind eye so you wouldn't have to change, or because of what others thought?

Transform Cycle

"It's better to live like a lion for one day than like a slave for a hundred years."

—Malala

There comes a time when the whispers of who we truly are get louder. When we start to realize that conformity hasn't made our dreams come true but instead has left us stuck, complacent, and unfulfilled. If we listen to the whispers and take action, the Transform Cycle begins. We begin to move from looking to the external world for all the answers to feeling from our internal source, trusting that we ourselves have what we need. We stop performing for others and start living for ourselves. We stop seeking external validation and start listening to the true desires of our hearts, embracing who we are inside, fighting to reveal who we really are, and finally exploring our purpose in life.

This is where the real journey begins.

———

By the time Alexis was five years old, I had done everything I was "supposed" to do. The good education? Check. The good job? Check. The marriage, the house, the happy daughter, the money, and the perfectly ornamented Christmas trees? Check. And yet I was stressed all the time, not feeling gratified about having finally made it, but empty and exhausted. I knew I did not want to have more kids, so I was left with the questions *What now?* and *Is this it?* in my mind. *This cannot be it,* I thought. *It is hollow, and not what I thought it would be.*

So I decided to remodel my house. I felt that if I fixed up my house, gave it a true makeover, then I would be made over too. After spending thousands of dollars on renovations—including the closet of my dreams, which, I admit, I now miss—I felt worse than before, and it certainly didn't improve my marriage. I was not made over. So I kept searching.

My mentor at Clark Nuber, Ned, had recently left to work for a real estate investment company. One day, out of the blue, he called me up and asked me to come work for him. That offer stopped me cold. I was on the partner track at my firm, on my way to the top, where I was certain I would finally be seen. Still, I considered it. *Should I take this leap onto a different path, one that might bring me more balance and happiness? Or should I stick to the known, even though it is causing me stress and confusion?*

After negotiations, Ned offered me a tax director position. The job came with the title, the money, and my name on the door. It seemed like a great move. I remember talking about this possibility with Eddie. "It could make things so much better," I said. "I could work less *and* make more money!"

His response? "If you take the job, I will never catch up to you."

That took the wind right out of my sails. But I knew deep down that I had to take the job, even if my husband did not support my decision. He was concerned about my making even more money than he did, but underneath that I think he was worried about how much I was going to outgrow him.

In 2007, I left my CPA job in public accounting. It was all I had known for most of my professional life. One of the ways I measured my worth was by how many hours I worked. Now I was choosing a different path. Little did I know, that was my marker of transformation. It was my moment of moving from the external to the internal, toward transformation.

I remember my first day at my new job. Previously, I had lived and worked in the suburbs and had not spent much time in downtown Seattle. Ned, who was now my boss, took me to lunch at Fado Irish Pub across the street from my new office. This may sound funny to those of you who live and work in the city, but for me, that foray was something of a culture shock. I was truly wide-eyed in wonder. I thought, *Where have I been all this time?* I felt so alive, and there was a part of me that felt more at home.

At my new job at Laird Norton, I was able to work less and create more space to do other things in my life. This meant that I could not avoid myself any longer. I had to look deeper.

For those of you who know me, you've probably noticed that I am a tenacious person. I achieve most things I set out to do. I have been an overachiever and overfunctioner all my life. But I had—and continued to have—an Achilles' heel: my body image.

I have been an athletic person my whole life, strong and sturdy. But being teased for my weight as a girl made a big impact on me. I internalized the same negative feedback that so many women receive for their size, and I struggled against my weight. The weight I'd gained during my pregnancy left me feeling even more insecure and uncomfortable. I decided to make a change.

About a year into my new job, my sister Holly started losing weight. One day she came over for a visit. As we chatted in the living room, Eddie complimented her on her new look. Later that night at the dinner table, he brought up Holly's weight loss and told me that I should weigh no more than one hundred forty pounds. I was twenty-five to thirty pounds away from that. I felt crushed. At the same time, I was ready to give a big fuck-you to that noise. And yet I did want to change my body, less for appearances' sake than to increase my fitness and energy levels. I wanted to *feel* better. I had been working out with my trainer and best friend, Dawni Rae, for about eight years and trusted her fully.

I realized that in order to change my body, I needed not only movement, but also lifestyle changes. I experimented with diets, and the super strict ones were torture. No carbs and few calories made me grumpy and miserable, and I knew I didn't want to live like that. The whole point was to feel better, not worse! Finally, after much soul-searching and with the help of Dawni Rae, I found a diet that worked for me. I had an ultrasound done to measure my lean muscle mass. From there, a food plan was generated based on my own muscle constitution. It was low-fat and low sugar, but I got to eat all the time! I got to eat the things I loved, and I felt my body transforming. I realized there is no one-size-fits-all diet plan. We each have to find what works for us and our bodies. I broke through a barrier that had existed in me my whole life, where I'd squashed the possibility and potential in my body. By freeing that potential, I felt empowered on a whole new level and saw myself in a new light. It was a catalyst for a massive shift.

I found new energy and confidence and began hip-hop dancing. This was a form of expression that exhilarated me, like something in me that had been suppressed was finally allowed to come out. I revealed parts of me that had always existed but were hidden. Though I loved hip-hop dancing, I was thirty-four years old, and it was hard on my body, so I needed to find a form of movement that was easier physically but just as expressive.

Enter hot yoga. For years, people had told me to try it. They "knew" I would love it. After my sister-in-law gave me a gift certificate to a hot yoga studio in Kirkland, I had no excuse not to try it.

I decided to go to a four-thirty class on a Sunday. I thought no one would be there on a Sunday afternoon. I walked into this tiny studio with no bathroom, no space for anything—it was just one dark, hot room, packed with sweaty, half-naked bodies. I was shocked. *What the hell is this?* I thought. We moved through a set sequence of twenty-six postures. The instructor was militant and stern. We were not allowed to take breaks, drink water, or leave the room. He kept telling us to go deeper, go harder, push. I fricking loved it! I was a type A CPA, and he was speaking my language. Though I had never practiced yoga, I felt like I did OK until he said, "You can at least do this one posture right!" I brushed it off and reveled in the sweat and exhilaration.

I immediately fell in love. To start, I went only once a week, but my mental well-being quickly began to shift. Those luxurious moments lying in *Savasana* quieted my mind and allowed insight to float to the surface.

I remember sitting on a bench with my aunt Yvonne, who often went to yoga with me, one day after practice. My hair was soaked with sweat, my little hot-yoga shorts and sports bra were drenched, and my mind and body were so, so relaxed.

"Yoga is changing me," I said. It wasn't just about my body—yoga was peeling back layers of my facade, revealing much of what I had long kept buried, opening my heart and my mind. I would never be the same again.

My aunt looked at me and smiled like a cat in a sunbeam. "It's changing me too," she said.

From then on, I began to see myself in a different way. My attachment to conventional standards started to crumble. All the "shoulds" no longer mattered so much. I wanted to be seen for me, not for what everyone else wanted me to be. I was ready to really see, to dive deep into the early messages that had shaped me and study them, shed them, and find what was true for me now. It was time to look within.

For years, I had been unhappy in my marriage. To be brutally honest, I don't think I was ever truly fulfilled in that relationship. This was not the first time I had this realization, but it was stronger than ever. I could no longer sweep it under the rug.

My two favorite aunts, Yvonne and Maureen, and I went for a getaway at Green Valley Spa in Utah. Yvonne's friend Ed came with us too. During our vigorous hikes, calming spa treatments, and quiet downtime, my spirit awakened, yearning to be free. I could tell there was something special happening with my aunt and her friend. My aunt was married to another man. She shared her struggles with me, and watching her inspired me to look at my own marriage. I knew I was unhappy and wanted more. I wanted to reclaim my life.

Back at home, I started having conversations with Eddie. I tried to express how I felt and my desire to be free to be who I was. This naturally caused distrust on his side. After eighteen years of being together, how could I have just shifted?

His immediate reaction was to assume I was cheating on him. He began sifting through my photos, hacking into my phone, and searching my internet history to try to make sense of things. In his mind, there had to be someone else. He was not willing to look within.

All that did was make me feel further away from him and more empowered to live who I was without those bonds, that cage that had held me back for so long.

Of course, he couldn't find anything—there was nothing to find—so he changed tactics. He saw my newfound confidence and, desperate to get the old, insecure me back, he started to put me down. One day he told me that our lack of good sex was because I didn't "feel" the same since having a baby. Ouch. Another day, as I was walking out the door to go to a yoga class, he said, "I just want the sixteen-year-old I fell in love with." Whoa. I knew in that moment that I'd outgrown him long ago.

Eddie's family joined in on his game. I'm sure they were scared about what might happen to their son and brother if he and I broke up. One night at dinner, I commented on his bad habit of running his fingers over his plate to mop up the last of his meal. So his mother picked up her plate and licked it from top to bottom.

I felt like they were trying to put me back in my place. The place I'd always been, the place that was comfortable for them. What if I had changed? Would that mean that they would have to change too?

Manifestation is a crazy thing. Eddie was convinced there was someone else. There wasn't. But after a few months of constant, fruitless conversations, of trying to work things out and getting nowhere, I started to become friendly with a colleague at another accounting firm. His name was Tim. I was his client. We had lunch a few times and discovered that we were both unhappy in our marriages. He was deep into therapy and encouraged me to go. I was tired of us trying to do it on our own. Nothing was changing. We needed help.

The first thing I asked our new therapist, May, was if she could fix our marriage. I knew it was broken. She looked at me with raised eyebrows as if to say, *Oh dear.* Eddie and I had several unhelpful sessions. He was good at telling people what they wanted to hear. I think he only agreed to go because he was worried about what I would say, worried about what the therapist might think of him. It was very clear to me that the marriage was over even before we started therapy. It had been over for months. We were barely talking, and we had no intimacy at all. Therapy was my one last failed attempt. I was done.

During this time of struggle in my marriage, and as I was transforming into the person I had been waiting for, I became good friends with a coworker named Rick. Rick had just gone through a terrible breakup and needed a friend. We would go to lunch, and he would cry on my shoulder. I would cry on his shoulder. It was a purely platonic relationship, and offered me so much more than a romantic relationship could have. He intoxicated me with his boldness and zest for life. He was passionate and knew what he wanted. That friendship lit a fire in me, inspired me to go after what I wanted too.

I became friends with Rick's best friend, Tom, too. Any time I could escape my house, the three of us went out. They were very attractive and charming, and a big part of me wanted to be seen by them, to be liked and accepted into their little club, the club of confidence and independence. I was blind to my need to be accepted by them because I was still transforming, but they became a critical piece of my journey.

Eddie knew about Rick and assumed he was the guy I was cheating on him with. Not true. But Rick did help steer me away by giving me permission to be who I wanted to be.

Rick's friend Tom started going to yoga with me. He loved it. Rick and I talked about my love for yoga during our lunches. I had been practicing for about a year, and we fantasized about the three of us owning a yoga studio. The low overhead plus our business skills plus my passion for yoga would be the perfect formula. To me, it was just a dream. That is, until one day when Rick strolled into my office with his charming grin.

"Chica, there's a spot in Queen Anne that used to be a Jamba Juice and would be perfect for a yoga studio," he said. I looked up from my computer. "Let's go check it out," he said.

I had never been to the Seattle neighborhood of Queen Anne. I was like, "Cool, let's get coffee afterward." Any excuse to get out of the office and hang out with my friend and dream, I was in.

The woman showing us the space was the daughter of the landlords. Neither Rick, Tom, nor I had ever owned a business before, and I don't think she took us very seriously. But the moment I walked into the space, something shifted in me. I recalled my memory of Celeste, the woman who read my palm and told me I was going to help a lot of people and do amazing things in life. This was it. The opportunity to transform my life, to find my purpose.

I knew I needed to do it. I needed to open this studio.

When I started talking about my plan to open a yoga studio, everyone thought I was going through an early midlife crisis. There I was with the husband, the house, the kid, the cars, the job, the success, the whole nine yards. They didn't know that my marriage was unraveling. From the outside, everything looked perfect. So what was I doing? Why would I want to destroy all that I had built?

But I had reached a breaking point. I wanted to be free. Free from it all. I wanted out: out of my relationship, out of my job, out of my life. I admit that there was even a brief moment when I wanted out of motherhood. I loved—and love—my daughter more than anything in this world, and simultaneously I wanted to be free of the responsibilities that come with raising a child. I wanted complete freedom from everything, from my life that felt so forced, so constraining.

One evening, after Andrea's wedding shower, where I'd had a few glasses of champagne, I met up with Eddie at his best friend's house for a Super Bowl party. I showed up buzzed and basically out of my mind. The whole night, I was draping myself over an ex-boyfriend and being completely belligerent. Eddie was embarrassed and rightly so. He went upstairs to the kitchen. I followed him and found him wallowing with his best friend and his best friend's wife.

"What's wrong with you?" I said, becoming hostile.

"I don't know, what's wrong with *you*?" he said.

"Don't be such a fucking pussy!" I yelled.

His friends' jaws dropped. *Who is this woman?*

That was the lowest point for me. I was desperate to move on, and Eddie would not budge. I believe I was subconsciously trying to sabotage our marriage so he would let me go. How could he stay with me after I talked to him like that? The humiliation would surely force his hand. But still he didn't leave.

I decided to go to Birch Bay with Andrea for one last pause before finally making the leap into ending things with Eddie. It was right before my birthday. Prior to the trip, I met up with Tim, the man from the other accounting firm who'd convinced me to go to therapy. We had become close. I felt like he saw me, and that I saw him. We were both so desperate for love and intimacy, so broken and unhappy. Our friendship had become flirtatious and he'd started sexting me. I'd responded, and we'd built up some serious sexual tension. So I knew meeting up with him would be risky. I did it anyway.

He was confident, so different from my husband, and very appealing to me. He took command. We had a cocktail downtown at the Arctic Club Hotel, a locale frequented by many of our colleagues. The lights were dim, and the mood was romantic. I was a little nervous but excited at the same time. My attention was on him. It felt dangerous, but I felt alive.

In the middle of our conversation, he leaned over and kissed me on the mouth. My heart started pounding. My desire for him was through the roof. I could feel the backs of my thighs tingle. He paid the bill, and we walked out of the restaurant and toward the elevator, then he whisked me into the stairwell. He grabbed my face and kissed me passionately. Then he pushed me up against the wall, lifted my skirt, opened his pants, and began fucking me in the stairwell of the Arctic Club Hotel. Someone could have walked through the door at any moment, but I didn't care. I let the moment completely swallow me up. For a woman who had been with only one man her whole life, who played by all the rules, and had only dreamed of these erotic moments but never experienced them, I was scared yet exhilarated and free for the first time. I had done something I never thought I would do; I acted impulsively and with sheer spontaneity. I left that stairwell and was changed forever.

I knew my marriage was over but still did not want to be judged, so I went on the weekend trip with Andrea but did not tell her what had happened with Tim. When I got home, I told Eddie that we were done and someone had to leave. We had no one to blame but ourselves.

Eddie refused to go, so I packed my bags and made an emergency appointment with my therapist. Then I stayed at a hotel for a few days. Those nights were some of the loneliest and most terrifying of my life. I'd been alone all along, yet I still did not know how to be alone. I reached out to friends, hoping they could distract me. I texted Tim but he didn't come. In the wee hours of the morning, I was left with only myself and my decision. I had no regrets; I just did not know what would happen next. I'd taken a blind leap hoping I would fly.

Eddie was still in denial. I think he thought I just needed a few days and I'd come back with my tail between my legs.

We met at the therapist's office, and I told my husband that I was not coming back. He didn't believe me. He rejected the idea of him staying with his parents. Instead, I ended up asking my mom and stepdad if I could stay with them. That was a truly humbling moment and a bad idea from the start. Since reaching adulthood, I had never asked them for help. I'd told myself that I would never go back like my sisters had, to fall back into the cycle of codependency. But I had nowhere else to go.

I took Alexis with me. I wanted her to know that I was not leaving her. She seemed to handle the situation quite well. She was highly intuitive, as most children are, and I think she was relieved to be free of the tension that had been palpable for so long at home. I'd tried to be open with her throughout the process so she would not be caught off guard when the time came. She stayed with me at my parents' the first three days, then she went back to her dad's. We decided to split time fifty-fifty right out of the gate.

During those first three days, I received a call from my friend Jane. She was originally my friend, but we'd become "couples friends" when our husbands met. She told me that Eddie had called them and seemed drugged or drunk, that he was hallucinating and talking about guns. I didn't know what to do. I didn't want to go to him because I was afraid. The next day, I mustered up the courage to see him. He said that "the devil got him." He was still talking crazy and had wild eyes, just as his sister had that time she'd climbed up on our roof. He reminded me of my father in his moments of alcohol-induced psychosis. It really scared me.

In our eighteen years together, I had never witnessed something like this, a "psychotic break" according to our therapist. I couldn't help but feel responsible; it was in that moment that I realized how much damage I had done to him in our marriage. His mother had coddled him, while his father had been hard and detached, domineering. I had coddled him, too, given him safety and stability, and now I was leaving. I grieved for him. I felt that I was failing him, that my taking control of everything had stunted him. Eddie had never had a chance to grow. He'd never been allowed to be himself. He'd never learned to fight for himself.

Now he couldn't handle what was happening. He was angry. There were so many family-of-origin issues and traumas that he'd never addressed to gain any insight or understanding around any of it.

I encouraged him to get help. Eddie resisted. He said he didn't need individual counseling. I'm sure that, underneath, he was just scared. Scared of being judged or criticized, scared of being vulnerable. It's much easier to pretend, even when it's not working. We want to be seen so badly, but we resist being seen because it makes us vulnerable.

I made it ten days at my parents' house. I'd arrived on my thirty-fifth birthday, which turned out to be the day that my maternal grandmother died. As you can imagine, it was not ideal. My mother was grieving the loss of her mother. I was grieving the loss of my marriage. We both needed support, and neither of us had anything to give.

My mom and stepdad got wasted every night. It was my worst nightmare. I quickly reverted to the ten-year-old girl who had to deal with the drunken instability of those who were meant to care for her. It certainly was not the safe haven I'd hoped for—in fact, the situation I'd left was better than the one I now found myself in.

On the ninth night, my mom and stepdad came home drunk and cornered me. "Leah," my mom slurred. "You should go on back to Eddie, give it another try."

"I can't, Mom," I said. I could feel a lump gathering in my throat.

"You're going to give up on eighteen years together just like that? Marriage takes work. Bob and I have had a great deal of tough times. What about Alexis?"

"I don't want to talk about this right now. And you're drunk," I said.

"Don't speak to your mother that way," my stepdad said. "What's wrong with you?"

"Leah, when are you going to quit being so angry with us? Why won't you forgive us?" my mom asked.

"Mom, I appreciate that you want to repair our relationship, but I am not in a place to work on it at the moment. I'm in the middle of a crisis and I have no room for that! We'll talk about it soon, just not now. Please."

"Well, hurry the fuck up because we're getting old," my stepdad said. "Bitch," he said under his breath as he puffed up his chest.

My mother fell to her knees.

"Lee," she wailed. "Won't you forgive me?" Big fat tears rolled down her face, smearing her mascara into two black lines on her cheeks. I simply sat there, not knowing what to do. I felt sorry for my mom, but at the same time, I thought it was selfish of her to ask this of me given the circumstances.

My silence infuriated my stepdad. "I don't know what planet you're from," he said. "What kind of person just sits there while her own mother's down on her knees begging for forgiveness! What the fuck is wrong with you?" My mom bawled louder. Bob kept going off, ranting about what a horrible person I was, pacing and turning red in the face. I was afraid he might come after me, so I finally ran off and locked myself in the bedroom. Just like I had in my childhood.

I left the next day to spend the weekend with friends. My mom called to tell me that if I was not willing to work on our relationship, then I was not welcome in her house. It was the first time I had ever asked for help, and she was threatening to kick me out. She had used that same scare tactic with my sisters, but I refused to budge. I was stronger than that. So I packed my bags and left with no idea where to go. Fortunately, Rick let me sleep on his couch for a few days while I searched for a place to live.

When we are on the right path, the universe sends us messages. Sometimes, they are crystal clear. I call these silver-platter gifts. My silver-platter gift came in the form of an ad on Craigslist—yes, Craigslist—in Queen Anne. Remember, I had only been to Queen Anne one time, to look at the potential yoga studio space. I didn't know that area at all. But the listing sounded appealing: it was a separate downstairs space, the upstairs occupied by a family who had a seven-year-old daughter, the same age as Alexis. Elation! I called the woman who'd placed the ad, and she told me that she had just given it away. Devastation. I thought it was a sign that it wasn't meant to be. I started searching again, but within an hour, the woman called back and said the other tenant had fallen through and the place was mine. Thank you, universe!

I met the family and got a tour of their beautiful home. My room would be in the basement. There were no windows, but it had its own bathroom and a little kitchenette. It was small and dark, but I did not care. Alexis and Jenna, the little girl who lived there, hit it off right away. We agreed that I would move in a few days later.

———

When I went to get my things from my parents' house, I found a letter on my bed. It was from my stepdad. The first line asked if I had a "hole in my heart." It went on in the same vein, saying that I was a hateful and resentful person, that I had no joy, that the bad things in my life were all my fault. I was accustomed to this kind of verbal abuse but would never get used to it. It cut deep.

Before, my therapist had called me Cinderella. She theorized that my parents' abuse stemmed from the deep resentment and envy they had for me. Now I realized that I needed to not only divorce Eddie but also separate from my mom and stepdad.

I was losing it all, by my own choice. It was incredibly difficult, but every fiber of my being told me it was not only better this way but also necessary to save my life.

We all experience trauma. A lot of trauma happens to us: disease, accidents, and circumstances beyond our control. But when we initiate the trauma with our own hands, it sticks. When we choose the trauma ourselves rather than having it happen *to* us, there is absolutely nothing more powerful than that. It is the highest level of courage.

Not only did I lose my marriage and relationship with my mom and stepdad, I also lost Eddie's family, a family I thought loved me. They wrote me off. They defended their son, which was natural. There was a strange twist, however: Eddie, my family, and Eddie's family all banded together. Eddie even started going to church with my parents. I felt like everyone was siding with him in order to somehow lure me back in. My resolve did not waver.

The only person who was there for me was my dad, now twenty years sober. Though he still lived in Spokane with his wife and their two children and was not in easy reach, he was just a phone call away. He was my phoenix that rose from the ashes. The one who was not there for me in my Primal Cycle was now my greatest ally. He never once hesitated. He encouraged me, told me I was doing the right thing when I had doubts. He stood by me even though he had a strong relationship with Eddie. It was the second time I felt true love from a parent. Again, it was my dad. I was forever changed by his support and love. I continued to lean on my aunts Maureen and Yvonne too. Yvonne was going through a similar conflict. We kept practicing yoga and searching for truth.

During this time, I was highly emotional, expressive, sexually charged, and active. I was running and practicing yoga. I danced all the time. Danced in my car, danced in my room in front of the mirror, danced in dance classes. Movement made me feel alive. It got me up off the floor when I was scared and broken.

The first night at my new place, after dancing my ass off in my room to Rihanna, my go-to transformation artist, I went for a run to get the lay of land. Little did I know, less than a mile away was the potential yoga studio space. Another silver-platter gift. I was moving toward my purpose, and the universe was guiding me.

Eddie and I were officially separated. I sought legal counsel. I quit going to marriage counseling and started going to individual counseling twice a week. I was like a blank canvas. Ready to express myself, experience vulnerability, and do deep work. I was looking for—and seeing—glimpses of the real me, and I was not about to stop. My therapist told me I was like a genie out of the bottle who was not going back in.

I continued to meet up with Tim from time to time. We were both separated from our spouses and seeking raw, unfiltered, uninhibited sex. We would book a hotel room for a few hours to take a romp in the sack. Or we would leave the office to meet in a dark parking lot just to get our hands on each other. The sexting was constant and beyond naughty. Once, I had an orgasm alone in my car just from the sexting. It was a crazy time. We were primitive animals that had been pent up for way too long and needed release. It was something I had been missing and now I was drinking it in.

The fact that I didn't get emotionally attached surprised me. In my inexperience, I assumed that I'd naturally feel a deep connection to any person I was intimate with. I figured I would want a relationship and fall in love. Yet with Tim I didn't. Did I care about him? Yes. Did I think of him when I was lonely? Yes. Did I want to be in relationship with him? Never. Over time, our encounters fizzled out with no drama. We simply reverted to being colleagues, albeit colleagues with a unique understanding of each other.

A few weeks after moving into my new home, the landlords accepted our lease proposal for the yoga studio. Rick, Tom, and I were in business! For the first time, I was making decisions based on what I wanted and who I wanted to be. Several months earlier, Irena, a highly intuitive coworker, came to me and told me she'd had a dream about me in which I was naked and watering a plant at its roots. She said that she had these dreams about people when they were about to go through something significant. Fast forward to five months later, and I am sitting in my therapist's office, describing my new place, my new business, and all the other crazy changes happening. I did not tell her about Irena's dream. To my shock, she said, "You just need to get planted so you can water your roots." Wow. I had embraced my nakedness, my vulnerability, and doors had opened. Everything was flowing in the right direction, I just had to be willing to surrender to what was happening within myself.

One of my favorite parts of therapy with May was analyzing my dreams. I am a vivid dreamer, especially when I am working on myself—when I'm "in the work." During that time,

I had a dream in which my mom was driving a car with Alexis, me, and my sisters in the passenger seats. The car spun out of control, and I tried to take the wheel. We went off the road and into an icy pond, then sank to the bottom. I got Alexis out first and then my sisters. I hesitantly pulled out my mom. Translation: The car represented my journey. The people in the car were important relationships I was working to save. The pond was my subconscious. It being icy represented my suppressed emotions. My trying to take the wheel was me trying to take control of my life. Sinking to the bottom signified that I was trying to get to the bottom of things.

I started to dig deeper into my own wounds now that the drama of the separation had settled a bit and I was out on my own. First off, I dove into my abandonment issues. These issues have been the bane of my existence. Fear of abandonment is my biggest trigger to this day. I realized that I had subconsciously chosen Eddie so that I could remain alone and abandoned without having to actually be alone. I wanted companionship, but I chose someone who did not see me and never would, and therefore I would always be inherently alone, empty, abandoned. I also wanted control. But my control was just a coping mechanism, an attempt to feel like I had power over my abandonment issues but which ultimately made me abandon myself. Oh, the irony. We humans are so good at sabotaging the very things we want the most, destroying ourselves while trying to protect ourselves.

Over the next few weeks, I saw Eddie every now and then for "family time," to determine if we could make amends or at least come together for the sake of our child. I knew I was done with our marriage, but there were parts of me that felt guilty for breaking up the family. I hear this all the time, that people stay in their marriage for the kids' sake. I can understand and respect that, but I was unwilling to stay for my daughter. I knew deep down that our divorce would be better for her, too, even though I was dismantling my family, not only my marriage but also my relationships with my parents and his. I struggled with the loss. So I kept trying. Each time Eddie and I came together, our communication was awkward and strained, and we failed to see a solution. That is what people do: Even when we know something's not working, we keep trying. It is called insanity. I had to break the insanity. I decided that I wanted a divorce.

Meanwhile, I had proceeded with the lease for the yoga studio. Then I got a call from the landlords. They had decided to drop us—apparently Rick and Tom were running the lease negotiations like a couple of bulldogs, and the landlords didn't want to deal with them anymore. I was devastated. I wanted that space so much.

It felt like everything was dying around me: my marriage, my nuclear family, my connections to my parents and Eddie's family, and now the studio and all the possibilities it might have brought. What could I do? I went to yoga. The teacher had a lesson that was unusual for the classes I attended early on. It was, "In order to be reborn, you must let everything die." In that moment, as my old life was dying, I was there waiting to be planted, watered, and reborn. I was not giving up, I was being given a new life.

I hadn't completely lost hope of getting that yoga studio space, so I took it upon myself to make one last attempt to rectify the situation. The landlords didn't know me, my passion, or the vision I had. I decided to write them a letter to show them me, my heart, and to kill them with kindness. They gave us back the lease. Love wins every time. I learned that early on in the process of transformation, and that lesson has carried me ever since.

———

With guidance from my therapist, I decided to start dating, casually. I felt like I needed to make up for lost time, and though I wasn't actively looking, I was ready to be open to it. Cue manifestation and the Law of Attraction.

I was out with my childhood friend Michelle, having a glass of wine at a bar. I'd known Michelle since I was twelve years old. She was my only friend who lived in the city, and she was all too happy to be my partner in crime in my new city life.

It was a chilly night. I'd just taken a sip of wine when in walked two men. My eye was instantly drawn to one-half of the pair, a lanky, six-foot-five African American man. It was like he fell from the sky right into that bar, into my life.

"That guy over there is exactly the kind of guy I am looking for," I said to Michelle.

She looked. "Him?" she asked.

I saw his friend lean over and whisper in his ear, and then he looked up. Our eyes met. He approached.

"Hi. Um, uh, I don't really know what to say," he said.

I gave him a kind smile and said, "You're doing fine."

His name was Martin. We had a nice conversation. He was not too forward, and I liked that about him. He gave me his number instead of asking for mine and walked me to my car. The ball was in my court. Would he be my first date?

Yes, he would. A week later we went out on a date. He took me to The Pink Door, an Italian restaurant near Pike Place Market. He ordered a Manhattan on the rocks, and I ordered a vodka soda. At dinner, I learned all about him. He was a film director and writer from North Carolina. He'd been in the navy for four years, two of which he'd lived off-base in Japan. He was forty years old; I was thirty-five at the time. He was beautiful, creative, outgoing, funny, worldly, and self-sufficient.

Our chemistry was off the charts. After sharing a plate of pasta, he walked me to my car. Not ready to end our evening just yet, I asked if he wanted to listen to music with me in my car. He did. Within moments, I was straddling him, and we were making out in the passenger seat. I knew I would see him again.

That night, I dreamed of Eddie showing up at my door, beaten to a bloody pulp by his own hand. It was a representation of what had happened and what was yet to come in his life and our marriage. It was time to file for divorce. But first I had to tell Alexis.

We continued to share custody of our daughter; she spent half the week with me and half the week with Eddie. Though Eddie was depressed, he seemed to be functioning normally without any episodes of psychosis (at least that I knew of).

It was my day to have Alexis. I picked my daughter up from school.

"Hey, Mom," she said, shrugging her backpack off her shoulder and placing it on the floor of the car. She got into the passenger seat and buckled her seat belt. "When are you coming home? When will we be a regular family again?" This was the first time she had spoken up. Before this, she was withdrawn and refused to talk about her emotions or acknowledge the situation. I started the car and pulled away from the curb.

"Your daddy and I aren't going to live together anymore. I love you, and I need you to know that none of this is your fault. It's just something that happened between your daddy and me."

She started to cry.

"Everything is going to be OK, sweetheart."

"I don't want to talk about it anymore." She turned her face toward the window.

"We have to keep talking. I know how hard this must be for you. It's hard for all of us. I've seen how you've taken our problems on, but it's not your job to take care of me or your dad. We're supposed to take care of you."

Eddie was depressed, and I was busy building my new life, which took a heavy toll on Alexis. On top of that, her dad would dig for information from her and make her promise not to tell me. She was internalizing a lot. But I was committed to being open and honest with her. That was going to be the backbone of my parenting going forward, I promised myself. No more holding back, censoring, or withdrawing based on my fear of Eddie's criticism. This would prove to transform Alexis's life as well.

A few days later, I met with Eddie at a coffee shop. I was planning to tell him that I was filing for divorce. My dad had had a conversation with him, in which he'd tried to facilitate some understanding and acceptance. Still, when I met with my soon-to-be ex-husband, I was certain he was going to resist, to say that we just needed to try harder, to get help, to do whatever it took. Instead, he said, "I know that you're done with our marriage. I'm ready to let you go."

I was shocked. Was this his last attempt to try to win me back? Did he think his releasing me would somehow scare me back to him? No way! I was free.

"OK," I said hesitantly. "Thank you, Eddie; thank you for letting me go." I began to talk about how to proceed with the divorce, and Eddie immediately started to worry about what people would think, what we should say, what we'd post on Facebook, and, most importantly, his not getting screwed in the divorce. He made it clear that he needed to be taken care of. Sigh. I listened to his demands, but there was no resolution at that point. It felt like he was backtracking.

We left together. Outside by the curb, Eddie asked me for one last kiss goodbye. I freaked out inside. It was like a complete stranger was asking me to kiss him. I decided to kiss him as a sign of gratitude for his letting me go. I turned to face him. He leaned in and kissed me. I stood my ground, neither giving in nor rejecting. He pulled away.

"Leah," he said. "I don't want this. I don't want you to go." I'd known the kiss was manipulation, that he was grasping for me and punishing me at the same time.

"I know, Eddie," I said. "But I do. It'll be good for us, for you, in the long run. I'm not the one for you anymore. You'll realize that someday."

I had to stop myself from skipping to my car. I was emancipated. I could not believe it. I was on fire. Completely uninhibited. That evening I went out with my friend Michelle to have a drink at a bar called Black Bottle. We met a guy there. After a few rounds, he invited us up to his penthouse in the Belltown neighborhood.

His place was amazing. It had a panoramic view of the city, amazing art on the walls, and a rooftop patio. He told us that he used to be a rock star in Los Angeles, then busted out his guitar and began serenading us. Next thing I knew, he was kissing me on the couch. He invited Michelle in, and then the three of us were kissing. I am telling you, I was going for it. It was a wild ride.

It was like the floodgates had opened and the water that had long been blocked was now gushing out. The next night, I went on my second date with Martin. We had the best time. I was committed to being totally honest and authentic. I told him I was going through a divorce and that I had a daughter. As if that's not enough to scare a guy away! But he stayed. He was grateful for my honesty. He simply wanted to know that the divorce was happening for sure and that there was no chance I would go back. He did not want to get involved with a married woman. I assured him it was happening.

At the time, he was working at Tully's Coffee's corporate office. He took me to their headquarters and showed me the movie he'd written and directed. It was brilliant. He was brilliant. I really liked him. In my dreams, my manifestations, he was the one. He was what I was searching for. But really, universe! I wasn't even divorced yet, and the universe sent me my dream man. It couldn't be. It was too good to be true. I'd resist. I'd hold him at arm's length. I would not get involved. At least, that's what I told myself.

A few days later, I got the keys to the new yoga studio space. It was official! Rick, Tom, and I were going to build a yoga studio. On top of that, the divorce papers had been served. My life was moving forward. I was moving closer to my truth. I danced in my room to "Rehab" by Rihanna on repeat all by myself that night.

Over the coming weeks, I was devoted to creating my new life. I spent some time with Martin. I told my boss about the yoga studio to get his approval and support. At the time, I had no intention of leaving my job. The studio was a place of my own, a place to practice, something to dedicate myself to because I wanted to, not because I thought I should. I planned to have a manager run it while I kept my "real" job. Or so I thought.

We began building out the space and I started hiring. I was going to be front of the house, the face of the studio. The guys would be back of the house. They were not passionate about yoga like I was. They were in it for the business, the money. What money? I will get to that later.

We were shooting to open on June 8, 2009, and already there was buzz around Queen Anne. It was April 11 when we started the build-out. We were ambitious!

It was during the ninety-day waiting period for divorce when Eddie told me he would not sign the papers. I had been living in the basement of the Craigslist house for three months. The Reynolds family was such a blessing to me. They helped me with Alexis, provided a safe and stable place to live, and we became lifelong friends, both the girls and the adults. You never know who you will meet on Craigslist! I am still so grateful for them.

Even though Eddie was dragging his feet, I decided to take the next steps in my new post-divorce life. I found a two-bedroom apartment in Magnolia, a neighborhood close to Queen Anne, in the same building as my childhood friend Michelle. Alexis would have her own room to paint pink, and she'd get to play with Michelle's dog. I would be paying the mortgage on my home, rent for this place, and the myriad costs of the studio. This was a financial stress but completely necessary. At the time, it seemed perfect.

One night before moving into my new apartment, Michelle and I were packing up my basement in Queen Anne when Eddie texted me a picture of us on our wedding day. In it we were so young, so full of hope, holding each other's hands like we meant forever. But it was a lie. And it only served to remind me of the cage I had been living in for the twelve years of our marriage. It was completely misaligned with who I was now. I felt nauseated and nervous. The feeling was familiar—it was the same feeling I had had when my dad was drunk, when I wasn't sure if he was going to hurt me or himself. I started to cry.

"Why are you crying?" Michelle asked. "Why are you so scared?"

I swallowed. "I just don't know what's going to happen. Everything's up in the air. When I was a kid and felt this way, I used to hide under the table waiting for the rug to be pulled out from under me."

"Why don't you talk to that scared little girl hiding under the table? Ask her what she wants."

I closed my eyes. I began to talk to Michelle as that little girl. "I want my mom. I want protection. I want love."

"Tell the little girl, 'I got this now. I don't need anyone because I have me. I am my protector. I have control of my life. I am OK. I love you.'" I repeated the words back as I cried the kind of cry where you almost can't breathe. Michelle paused. "How old is the little girl hiding under the table?"

"Seven." Seven is a powerful number for me. I was born on the seventh. I was seven when I went through a big family trauma. At this time, Alexis was seven, and I was thirty-five, a multiple of seven.

The numerology and synchronicity of this meant a lot to me. I had to face this little girl who had been me, who was the same age as my little girl. I could not live in fear anymore, and I would not let my daughter live in it either. It just so happened to be the eve of Easter, the holiday of resurrection and rebirth. I felt reborn in that moment.

I set significant boundaries with my parents: They asked me over for Easter. I declined. This was huge. For the first time, I was not with my family for the holiday. I grieved the loss of that tradition but felt free from the burden of it and the dysfunction it always brought to the surface. I was getting good at making decisions based on my own health and truth, and that meant saying no.

After that, I got Alexis to agree to go to therapy. I knew she was struggling, and I was determined to have her get help earlier than I had. Therapy did so much for me, and I wanted her to have an outlet too.

I was worried about how Eddie was parenting. My therapist assured me that Alexis would be fine as long as she had one healthy parent and therapy. I took her referral and found a therapist whom Alexis liked. I often wonder what it would have been like if I'd had a therapist at a young age. Of course, wishing things had been different is a waste of time.

I had to get my things from the house in Bothell in which Eddie and I had made a home for nearly twelve years. I was willing to give him almost everything. In the process of finalizing our divorce, it had been decided that I would give him the house, fifteen hundred dollars per month in spousal support for two years, and child support each month, even though our parenting plan was split fifty-fifty. I was not done taking care of Eddie. This was frustrating, but I did it for my daughter, and honestly, I had not broken the cycle of overfunctioning yet. I wanted Alexis to stay in the house she'd grown up in and at her school. I wanted her to feel safe and secure. That was the cost.

Mostly what I wanted was to start over. Michelle and my sister Holly came with me to what had been my house, when Eddie was not there. I felt like I was breaking into someone else's home. I did not want much—only some clothes, some items with sentimental value, and my wedding ring. I had taken it off and had not been wearing it for months. Eddie rationalized that it was about my weight loss, but the truth was that I had not been wearing it because I no longer felt married to him.

I left all the furniture except the bedroom set. The bedroom set had been custom made, and I had paid for it. I left the mattress on the floor. That moment still haunts me. I imagine Eddie coming home to find my things gone and the mattress on the floor; the image breaks my heart. I know it must have been so hard and hurtful to him. I did not do everything right. I was transforming. Sometimes, my story—my pain, my needs—trumped all others. I was consumed by my escape from my lonely, caged-up life and my new taste of freedom, and I could not see clearly all the time. I am sorry for that. If I could go back, I would do things differently.

The next time I saw Eddie, while dropping off Alexis, he asked me why I'd taken the wedding ring.

"Because it's mine," I told him. "What would you do with it, anyway?"

"I would put it back on your finger," he said. I felt nervous and scared, cornered. He followed me to my car, begging me for forgiveness. I got in my car, but he would not let me close the door. He leaned in and grabbed me.

"Please, Eddie, let me go," I pleaded. "I don't blame you for all of this. It's not your fault or my fault. We just aren't good together anymore." We were both so unseen. The difference was that I was not willing to be unseen anymore. Finally, he let go, tears in his eyes, and stepped away from the car.

I bawled as I drove away. I was officially gone. The person I'd been was gone forever.

Marc, the man I'd met during the bachelorette weekend in Las Vegas, emailed me out of the blue. This was the same Marc whom I'd nearly left Eddie for seven years earlier (there's another seven). Well, actually, I had been thinking of him a few days before he emailed. Manifestation again.

By this time, Martin and I had been dating casually. We were sleeping together too. I was still trying to keep him at bay, but he was really into me. He told me he loved me early on. I was not willing to go there yet. Honestly, I was hung up on the fact that we got together so soon after I'd left my marriage. I kept wishing I could have met him two years down the road, so that I'd have had some time to experience single life and do my personal work. I wasn't ready to commit to an exclusive relationship after being in one for so long. But my therapist told me that the universe works in perfect order. Now I believe her, but at the time, I resisted.

I was candid with Martin about being contacted by Marc. There was a part of me that felt like I needed to explore that. Why would he reenter my life after all this time, and with perfect timing too? Martin told me to explore it. So I did. I called up Marc, and he asked me to come to Los Angeles. That's when his *wife* picked up.

"What the hell?" she said.

I never heard from Vegas Marc again. Martin won, and not by default. He won by honoring my truthfulness and allowing me the space to explore, and having the patience to wait for me. He continued to support my growth, and he introduced me to the book *The Four Agreements: A Practical Guide to Personal Freedom* by Don Miguel Ruiz. That book changed my life.

Eddie, on the other hand, was not giving me the space I needed, nor honoring my truthfulness or supporting my growth. In fact, he was threatening to contest my custody of Alexis, in a desperate attempt to prolong the divorce and scare me into submission. Though I was saddened and disheartened, I refused to back down. I recognized it for the empty threat it was and prepared myself to play hardball. If he followed through on contesting custody, it would become a battle of proving who the better parent was. We would have to air all our dirty laundry, which was Eddie's worst nightmare. And so it never came to pass.

Meanwhile, Tom, Rick, and I had agreed on the name hauteyoga Queen Anne for our yoga studio. We had the logo and website, and we were in the final stages of the build-out. Like most construction projects, it was late and way over

budget. Since Rick, Tom, and I were all in the financial business, we did the formation paperwork ourselves, without
attorneys and accountants. We had bootstrapped the business,
meaning we had all contributed capital. Nothing was financed.
I had drained my 401(k) to invest in the business, and we had
no working capital left. This was 2009, in the middle of the
real estate crisis. Banks were definitely not giving loans.

People thought we were crazy to open a business during
that time. I was used to that—people thought I was crazy for a
whole lot of other things too. During moments of stress, Tom
reminded us that the Rockefellers had had their biggest success
during the Great Depression. No risk, no reward, we told ourselves. I had already lost so much: my marriage, my family, the
life I'd worked so hard to create. And I was still breathing. So I
knew I would be OK if this failed too.

I had found a studio manager, but I needed teachers. I was
not a teacher yet. I had only practiced at one studio, taking
classes that involved doing the same twenty-six poses every
time. The studio I practiced at was in the suburbs, what locals
called the Eastside. It was a little behind the times out there,
whereas in the city, there was more variation in yoga styles.
Back then, there were only a handful of well-known studios in
the area, and I was a little naive. I knew business, not the yoga
industry. Still, I reasoned, I'd found a home on Craigslist, so
why not teachers?

That makes me laugh now. I would never in my wildest
dreams do that today. But that was where I was at. Even so, I
was a little wary that people would not take me seriously since
I was not a yoga teacher myself. I was doing it backward and
feared that people might not trust my abilities and know-how.
Fortunately, I got some good hits, mainly from people moving
to Seattle. And the woman whom Rick was dating loved her
yoga teacher and begged her to talk to me.

Her name was Anne Marie, Anne for short. Anne was well known in the industry and hesitant to talk to me because she didn't know me and she didn't like hot yoga. Rick's girlfriend convinced her to anyway.

I will never forget the day I met Anne. I was sitting in Starbucks drinking my soy latte, and I see this woman—who was pushing forty years old, in pigtails, wearing a fluorescent pink backpack with a giant yoga mat sticking out the back—walk in the door. I waved her over. She wore thick black eyeliner and a nose ring. I was dressed in business attire. She was on the defensive.

"Here's what I'll do," she said. "I will teach for you a maximum of two classes a week. The classes need to be during prime time because I want them full. And I won't teach in a room that is too hot, and I want to be able to monitor that."

When she was done, I said, simply, "OK."

She looked at me, perplexed.

"Do what you want," I said. The thing was, I had just been set free. I was learning to be who I wanted to be and practicing my own truth, and I was not about to tell someone else how to be. I've stuck to that principle ever since. "Teach how you want to teach," I tell my teachers. "Offer the world your gifts."

"I don't want you to be me," I told Anne that day. "I want you to be you." How could she say no to that?

"Well, OK then." She accepted.

"You got it," I said. I had Anne, a rock-star yoga teacher already established in Seattle, and my team of teachers from Craigslist. We were ready.

We held our grand opening party on June 6, 2009. I did not invite my mom or stepdad. My dad, who lived in Spokane, was unable to attend. But all our friends came. Rick's parents surprised him with a visit from California to show their support.

To me, the experience felt very disjointed. Though the studio was beautiful and I was excited and proud of our accomplishment, I no longer felt close to most of my old crew. They didn't really know me anymore. They all got drunk, and the photos they posted on Facebook did not reflect what I was trying to do. Fortunately, I had a few key supporters in my aunt Yvonne and Dawni Rae. They helped remind me who I was.

Martin came to the opening too. No one knew we were dating. My high school friends knew me only with Eddie, and our divorce was not yet final, so I felt the need to keep hiding that part of my life. Martin pretended to be the mayor of Seattle and gave me the key to the city. What a charmer. It was fun to watch the girls swoon over him. I was proud he was mine, even secretly.

Two days later, the doors of hauteyoga Queen Anne officially opened. I took the day off work to help my manager "tame the crowds." Again, in my naivety, I thought, *Build it and they will come.* The studio I practiced at was tiny, dark, and dirty, and always packed. I thought for certain that if I created a high-end space—including a bathroom—people would come in droves. Thank goodness for that naivety, because had I known what was really going to happen, I would have never opened the studio.

There were five classes on the schedule opening day. Three people came to the first class, five to the second, one to the third, three to the fourth. Rock star Anne pulled in a whopping thirteen for the last class of the day. Mind you, the room could hold thirty-five students.

There were thirty-two classes that first week, with a grand total of seventy-five students. That is an average of two and a half people per class!

Tom and Rick panicked. They said, "We are going to go bankrupt! We are going to be bums! We will soon be living on the side of the road!" It was a little dramatic, but the fear was real. And people who are afraid don't always think straight. Tom and Rick blamed me for the lack of attendance. Since they were in the back of the house, they could see only numbers, while I, in the front of the house, saw potential. I saw the community that would form, made up of motivated people hoping to live better. I saw gratitude and the difference the classes were making for the few who attended. Not for one second did I think the studio was going to fail. I had my vision, my mission, and glimpses of my *dharma*, my purpose. I was not going to give up.

Within a few months, Tom wanted out. In our partnership agreement, which we still had not signed, we'd planned that I would eventually buy him and Rick out. They were in it for the investment, and we all knew that three owners could not make a living off the business. My hope was that within a few years I'd be able to own it outright. But the plan changed from two or three years to just a few months. At the time, Rick and I were working well together. He and Tom often played against each other, but ultimately they had each other's backs. And when all three of us were working together, blame usually fell on me.

Anne and Rick had become close too. He recognized her knowledge of the industry and knew she could be a game changer. He proposed that we make her our director of yoga. In that role, she would be more invested, better able to take on more classes, and motivated to help foster more business. But after she was appointed, Tom and Rick started to play her against me too.

I felt like they constantly questioned my every decision, and I was always trying to prove myself to them. The relationship that had once felt so inspired turned sour. I had left one bad partnership and entered right into another one. All I could do was learn and try to maintain my truth.

But things just kept getting worse. We were out of money and needed additional capital, which I had to borrow from a friend. We took drastic measures and cut a bunch of classes from the schedule and cut the instructors' pay. I will never forget making those calls to the instructors to tell them that they were going to be paid less than agreed upon. I am grateful that all but one teacher stayed.

I had to let my manager go. We were paying her forty thousand dollars to run the studio! What were we thinking? I stepped in and took on her responsibilities. I started working at the front desk as much as possible. I would wake Alexis up at five-thirty in the morning and bring her to the studio with me so I could check in students. She would curl up in the corner and go back to sleep.

I was still working a demanding full-time job as a tax director. I slept three or four hours a night for nearly a year. People told me it was not sustainable, that I would get sick. But I had so much adrenaline, a fire, an internal knowingness that it would all be worth it. I knew I could dig deep. I knew I had the strength to endure.

Somehow, I found time to spend with Martin. He was my escape, my fun, my soft place to land. On days I didn't have Alexis, I would open the studio, go to work for eight or nine hours, go back to the studio, then meet up with Martin around nine or ten at night. He always had a cocktail waiting for me. I was not much of a drinker, but during that time, we were going out a lot. He showed me the city, taking me to a new place practically every night. We would stay up until three in the morning doing the things that people falling in love do, then the alarm would go off just a few hours later. Each morning, I would sit on the end of the bed, and he would breathe with me and say, "You can do it."

I surrendered to the fact that I was falling in love with him and stopped pushing him away. We had so much in common, and we could not keep our hands off each other. We had sex all the time and everywhere: in the car, on the kitchen counter, even on the conference table at Tully's headquarters. His hands were up my skirt before we could even make it in the door. Every day with him felt like Christmas morning.

Martin was patient and thoughtful, and most of all, he did not try to clip my wings. He was my biggest supporter and encouraged me to be my best self. I had never felt love like that before. To me, it was worth the risk of being judged for getting into a relationship so soon after my divorce, and for being in a relationship with an African American man.

I had never dated a black man before, and I worried about what people would think. That sounds terrible, and I cringe thinking that I ever even cared, because it is so far from where I am now, but it's true. Racism was—and is—alive and well, even in our liberal bubble of Seattle. But remember, I was new to the city. I'd lived in the homogenous suburbs. I struggled with what my friends and family might think. Especially when the first friend I told responded with, "How black is he?" *Really?* Then I reminded myself that no one gave a shit about who I was dating. And if they did, that was none of my business. Plus, they had their own stuff to worry about. They weren't thinking of my dating life.

I made, and make, mistakes when it comes to dealing with race. I am a white woman with good intentions, which are often not enough. I used to tell Martin that I did not see his color. I thought I was being loving and kind, but he got offended. I didn't understand why. Later, I learned that for him to feel seen, I had to see that part of him and the long history and daily trials that came with it. I get it now.

———

After a few months of dating, it was time for Martin to meet Alexis. My daughter tended to be shy, so when I introduced her to Martin in the children's books section of Barnes and Noble, she clung to me for dear life. In fact, she wanted nothing to do with him, this man who was not her dad. Her dad was home, sad and wanting the family to be together again. There was a long road ahead.

Then I was late. Yes, I'm talking about my period. Martin and I were having unprotected sex. I know, I know.

I had just gotten back from a trip when I told Martin that I thought I might be pregnant. He was calm. He did not push for answers. We immediately hopped in the car and drove to a Rite Aid near his condo to get a pregnancy test. We had to wait until morning to take it, and let me tell you, I did not sleep well that night.

I woke up at four in the morning and went into the bathroom in Martin's bedroom. It took my eyes a moment to adjust to the light. I left the bathroom door cracked so Martin could hear me if I needed him. He woke up and waited quietly on the edge of the bed. My hands shook as I opened the box, took out the test, and unwrapped it. *Please,* I thought as I peed on the little plastic stick. Then time slowed, I felt dizzy—I swear, every second of those five minutes waiting for the results felt like an hour.

It was positive. From my seat on the toilet, I collapsed onto the floor, wailing. Martin picked up my rag-doll body and carried me to bed. He held me and told me it would be OK. How could I have let this happen?

There was only one option for me. Honestly, I didn't even need to think about it. By nine o'clock, I was at the doctor; by two o'clock, I was having an abortion. I was six weeks pregnant. The doctor asked me if I wanted to see the monitor, and I turned my head away. I completely detached. The procedure took less than five minutes.

Martin went with me. He was supportive but without a doubt a bystander. I knew he wanted a baby, a child of his own, but I wasn't open to having a conversation about it. There was no way I could have a baby. My divorce wasn't final, my daughter was struggling, and my business was foundering. My body, my choice. I didn't feel guilt or shame (or so I thought), though I did ask for forgiveness in a prayer to God. I also got an IUD the next week—no way was I going to go through that again. I told myself I would never speak of it. I knew I made the right choice, but I felt like it was no one's business. It was like I was pretending it never happened.

A few more months went by. I dreamed of an old freezer. It was stuck in place, and try as I might, I couldn't move it. I felt suffocated, thinking someone or something was inside. Then I realized that Eddie was the freezer, and I couldn't move or change him. I was suffocating. I was waiting to be released once and for all. *Please let me go,* I begged.

In early October 2009, eight months after the divorce papers were served, I got a call from my attorney. Eddie signed! *Why the change of heart?* I wondered. *He must have met a girl.* That was the only way he would have budged. He needed a replacement. Whatever the reason, it didn't matter. Whatever it took to close that chapter was fine with me.

A few nights later, I was sitting with my daughter and Michelle in the living room. I was trying to play it cool, but finally my curiosity got the best of me.

"Does your dad have a new girlfriend?" I asked.

She blushed. "Yeah," she said.

"Oh," I said, my voice rising half an octave. "What's her name?" Alexis hesitated. I waited, perplexed.

Eventually, she replied, "Leah."

Gulp. *What?* I tried not to freak out. *Her name is Leah. The first person he meets, her name is Leah.*

Eddie married that Leah within the year. I call her Leah Number Two. She reminded me of the old me. She handled things, held it all together. She was the breadwinner, climbing the corporate ladder.

I continued to grow; the yoga studio continued to grow. I continued with my therapy, and classes started to fill. Within six months, we were showing a profit. As I revealed my true self, my purpose started to appear. It became clear to me that I had outgrown my job. I did not belong there anymore. I felt like my coworkers no longer understood me, and that I no longer understood them. I was confined, made to conform to the standards of corporate America. My look started to change—I wore rings on most of my fingers, little to no makeup, and edgier clothing. My demeanor changed too. I felt like people were uncomfortable around me. They knew I'd opened a yoga studio, and some people were interested, but most were not. Were they afraid I was going to start chanting *om* during Monday morning meetings?

Rick had been fired right before we opened the studio, so that office alliance was gone. My relationship with my mentor, Ned, started to feel strained. I knew I did not want to be there anymore.

It wasn't just work. Eddie and I had had many of the same friends since junior high, so naturally I lost some friendships because people took his side or the change made them uncomfortable. I suspect that many took it personally.

The loss of one friend in particular made me sad. Rebecca was married to Eddie's best friend. We'd grown up together, been high school sweethearts together. In our adult lives, we saw each other frequently, and we got together on New Year's Eve for many years. She and I understood each other. We each had similar struggles with conformity, and we leaned on each other during the hard times. But during the divorce, she stood by her husband, who stood by Eddie. There was no goodbye. I missed her and hoped she would be in my life again someday.

Many other friends stuck by me, but then I was the one who became distant. I had a harder and harder time going back to anything related to my old life. My friends invited me to our usual outings and parties, and I declined. It wasn't that I didn't love them anymore, it was that I could not identify with the person I had been when we'd built our friendships. Slowly but surely, most of them stopped extending the invitations. Michelle and Andrea still hung on, but something began to shift there too.

In February 2010, I went by myself to a yoga retreat in Sayulita, Mexico. It was a life-changing experience for me. It had been about a year since I'd left my house, marriage, and families, opened my business, and met Martin. I had been through so much and a lot had changed.

I intentionally used this trip as an opportunity to process all that I had been through, to be alone and enjoy the new person I had become. I was successful in terms of those objectives, but I also got an insight that I wasn't expecting: I saw where there were gaps in my growth, where I was repeating self-destructive cycles.

As I mentioned, my therapist encouraged dating but had told me not to get into a committed relationship for one year after the dissolution of my marriage. Since I was in an early phase of the Transform Cycle, the odds of repeating unhealthy patterns and self-destructive cycles were extremely high. I knew her advice made sense, but I didn't follow it. I was in a full-on committed relationship with Martin.

But during that trip to Sayulita, an abandonment and fear trigger reared its ugly head. Martin retreated from me. I called him and called him, left voicemails, did everything I could to reach him with the spotty cell service in town. He just didn't respond. I was worried. Was he punishing me for going on this trip without him?

Then I came to the conclusion that he'd abandoned me. Holy hell, I'd done it again. I'd chosen someone who would abandon me. All the pain of my childhood trauma hit me as though my dad had left yesterday, or my mom had just told me that she wasn't going to come home as I hid under the dining room table, or Eddie had retreated to his shed. This time, however, I was no longer the same person. I wasn't dependent on emotionally immature people caught up in their own drama. I'd chosen someone who was self-sufficient, independent, and emotionally attuned. And then he, too, left me in the dark, alone and blindsided.

Martin had his own brand of abandonment issues. His father had gotten involved in an extramarital affair and left the family when Martin was young. They'd been wealthy, but when his dad left, all the money went with him. Martin went from riches to rags, and fatherless to boot.

After that, his dad would promise to go see him and his brothers and then never show. His mom worked two jobs just to keep them fed. Martin's birthday is close to Christmas, so as a kid, he never had his own party. One time, his mom forgot his birthday entirely.

Martin had an unstable childhood similar to mine, and like me, he learned early to do everything on his own. We were both good at being alone, taking control so no one could let us down, and being stubbornly independent. So it's no surprise that we got into power struggles over who was more invested in the relationship, who was more present, who was needier, and who could withhold more. I'd played hard to get, he'd chased me, and now I was caught. And he knew it.

When I got back from Sayulita, I anxiously waited for him to pick me up at the airport, thinking he would be excited to see me. My heart clenched as he pulled up to the curb in the terminal. He parked and got out, but he wouldn't look at me. He was quiet, like a parent giving the silent treatment as punishment. I got in the car and started to cry, and we fought the whole ride home. Somehow, I found myself asking him for forgiveness for going on that trip.

Eventually we made up, but I knew this was far from over. Sure enough, Martin started going dark more often. I would not hear from him for days. It killed me.

Not only that, but his drinking problem became glaringly apparent. He drank almost every day. I hadn't noticed it at first because we were in a fun fantasy land, going out every night, seeing the city. I was intoxicated with pleasure and the exploration of my new freedom. I simply did not want to see it.

Once I realized that, I started to pull away. There was no way I could be in a relationship with an alcoholic after what I'd been through. I started making new friends and hanging out with Rick and Tom more. There was a codependency thing happening with them too. Even though they were hard on me about the business, they were still showing up for me in my personal life. They liked me better when I was down. They knew how to fix me up.

I slowed down communication with Martin, and unsurprisingly, he came running.

I was asleep in my bed when I heard a key turning in my apartment door. I pulled the sheet up to my chest to cover my naked body. My bedroom door swung open.

"What the fuck, Martin?" I screamed. "What are you doing here?"

His face was full of fear. He was panting in anger. "Where have you been, and why aren't you returning my calls?" he asked. Oh, the double standard. It was OK for him to go dark, but the moment I didn't answer his calls, he barged into my apartment?

"I don't want to be with you anymore, Martin," I said, my voice trembling. "You're up and leaving, the drinking, and now this? I can't do it anymore."

Suddenly he changed his tune. "Please, baby, no. Stand in the fire with me. I promise I will be better," he pleaded. I stayed.

During this same time, Michelle, the childhood friend who had seen me through the first part of my transformation, started to get possessive. Really possessive. If I did not call her after therapy and give her the lowdown immediately, she would psycho-call me, calling me over and over until I picked up. She needed to be involved in every part of my life. She would even hang out with Martin sometimes when I wasn't around.

Other friends had warned me about her potential problems with codependency, but I hadn't recognized it until now. Michelle also had maternal abandonment issues. Her focus on me was not real love—dependency takes rather than gives. Love gives.

One day, I decided to not answer her call. We still lived in the same building, and when Alexis and I got home that evening, shortly after arriving and taking a shower, there was banging at my door and Michelle screaming at us to let her in.

"It's OK, sweetie," I said to Alexis as I stood there with a towel wrapped around my head. I opened the door to find Michelle crazy-eyed and desperate.

"Why didn't you answer your phone?" she screamed.

"I was in the shower!" I said.

"You have to answer your phone. I *need* you to answer your phone," she maniacally repeated.

My daughter started crying. I was scared. I felt like we were in a scene from *Single White Female.*

Our decades-long friendship ended that day. I moved out a few weeks later to a place near the studio.

Martin and I had been dating a little over a year when his mother came to town. I'd known she was arriving, but for ten days I didn't hear from my boyfriend.

Finally, the day before his mother's departure, Martin called me and invited me over to meet her. I was not sure how I felt about going to meet her on her last night, and I was angry at Martin, but I decided to go. At his condo, Martin greeted me at the door and guided me into the living room, where his seventy-year-old mother sat in his recliner. She was short and round, wearing glasses and red lipstick. I sat down on the sofa and we chatted, mostly small talk. She was very pleasant, but I could feel an undertone of possessiveness of her son. During that conversation, she mentioned the gathering they'd had the other night. I learned that Martin had thrown a party during the ten days he'd gone dark. All his closest friends had come over to eat his mom's famous fried chicken with all the fixings. Everyone but me.

How could he not invite the person he loved? I was crushed. That feeling went all the way down to the deepest part of me, the part that felt wholly unwanted, unseen, and abandoned. Martin and I went into another room to talk and started to get into it, in that whispered shouting you do when you're so angry but trying to hide it. I stood up to leave, and he literally pushed me out the door.

"It's over," I said, then stormed off without saying goodbye to his mom. I got in the car and slammed the door. I was half-way down the block before he called me. I picked up.

"What?" I said.

"Leah, please come back."

"No. I am so done, Martin!" I cried.

"Please! I'm sorry, I don't want to lose you," he begged.

"Why? I am so sick of feeling like this." I felt defeated.

Finally, Martin managed to convince me to come back (again). His mother had gone to bed, and he and I talked until three in the morning, trying and failing to work it out. In my mind I was plotting to come by when he was at work the next day and get my stuff. It was an interesting tug-of-war of me wanting to leave (abandon) him before he could leave (abandon) me. It was the battle of who was going to leave whom first.

The relationship was not healthy, and there was no way I could stay in it any longer. I had worked too hard on myself to let someone treat me like that.

I truly planned to leave. But the next day I got a call from Martin. "I lost my job," he said.

I could hear the fear in his voice. How could I leave him after that?

I talked it over with my therapist. She urged me to leave him. She believed that he did not know how to be in a couple. Other than being in a brief marriage, he had been alone since the age of eighteen. "He doesn't know how to do the 'we,'" she said. I wasn't sure I knew how to do it either. I stayed.

For Thanksgiving, Martin (who was still unemployed), Alexis, my aunts Yvonne and Maureen, and I went to Bodega Bay, California. It was my one last attempt to see if there was hope for Martin and me, or so I thought. Immediately after we arrived, he withdrew. He tried to connect with Alexis, who wanted nothing to do with him. I'm sure she could tell that I was unhappy, just as she knew when I was unhappy with her dad. Later, Martin yelled at me about it, saying that she did not respect him. He was never around, so how could they build a relationship? How could he expect to have my daughter's trust?

Even after that, I still tried to get close to him. I would try to kiss him, but he pushed me away.

Then, at Thanksgiving dinner, he told Alexis to eat her vegetables. This is a bold parenting move, one that he had not earned. She began to cry. He was embarrassed. For the next two days, he retreated from me, with little to no communication. One late morning, I was practicing yoga in front of the bay window in our room. Beyond were the ocean and sky, the gray clouds and the giant waves crashing onto the shore. It was peaceful and serene. Martin sat in the corner in a rocking chair, drinking Jameson whiskey. In that moment I knew it was over. For the first time, I was not only hurt but also simply no longer attracted to him.

When we boarded the plane to go home, I looked him in the eyes and shook my head gently, and he knew.

Back in Seattle, we sat alone in my car outside my house.

"It's over," I said.

"No, Leah," he said. "Please. I'll . . . I'll get help, deal with my issues. OK? Just please don't go. I cannot handle losing both you and my job at the same time."

"I can't do this anymore," I said.

He didn't say anything, just looked out the windshield. It was a blustery afternoon, the wind blowing wet leaves down the street. "What if we had some time apart but didn't break up? I can't bear to think of you with anyone else."

"No," I said. "That won't work. I need to fly solo for a while, to be truly on my own." Martin did not like it, and I wasn't sure he would honor my space. So I changed the locks.

———

Running a small business is no easy feat. It is a 24/7 job, a labor of love. If you aren't passionate about what you are doing, then forget it. It is not for the faint of heart. You need to be willing to sacrifice sleep, money, time, and relationships. You have to be willing to jump out of bed or leave a party at the drop of a hat to fix the broken toilet and mop the floor.

Most importantly, you have to be willing to deal with people. The yoga industry can be a touchy-feely industry. Many people who are dealing with injury, trauma, and hardship come to the studio. And I carry, facilitate for, and am present with—or hold space for—these people, whether they are students, teachers or employees. I realized that I have a real knack for connection and for building community. It's actually not all that complicated: I ask for and remember people's names, always have a smile ready, and take a genuine interest in their lives. At the end of the day, we all just want to be ourselves and feel welcome and connected. I've always loved bringing people together but never had the right platform. Until I opened the studio.

Dealing with teachers and employees was a whole other ball of wax. I paid my employees minimum wage, so I had to work extra hard to find the right ones. Fortunately, there was a college down the hill, so there were lots of great young people to choose from.

I quickly learned that teachers are human, and that they often teach from their own mistakes, of which they—we—make many. Leading and coaching teachers became one of the most challenging parts of running the business. But I was committed. My partners were not. They wanted me to buy them out. By this time, I knew I wanted to leave my corporate job at some point, so I was ready to proceed.

Anne and I got closer as she began to lift Rick's veil of charm. She started to realize that much of what Rick said about me was a lie. She was a good person, fighting her own demons, and she was coachable. She was open to hearing my feedback and making shifts to facilitate her own growth. She had a wide-open heart. She just needed to trust me. She became a confidante and friend to me and was truly a pivotal person in growing hauteyoga in its early stages. Her classes were always full, and she brought me knowledge of, and insight into, the industry. I started to grow my other teachers to try to level out the playing field. If I was going to buy out my partners, I wanted to be on solid ground first. I also knew that I needed to be a teacher too. I wanted to be a teacher, not only for business purposes, but because I believed I would be good at it. I wanted to help people in the classroom, not just at the front desk.

Apparently I was due for another silver-platter gift from the universe, because I received a résumé from a woman named Katrina, who owned studios in the Chicago area and was moving to Seattle to follow her love. Her résumé was impressive and, to be honest, a little over the top. I was skeptical. She called me at the studio one day and we talked for a long time. I was happy to discover that we were on the same page and her philosophies aligned with mine. And that she wanted to introduce teacher training to hauteyoga.

"I'll teach you to be a teacher," she said. I was overjoyed at the possibility of learning to become a teacher in my own studio.

I hired her, and I'm so glad I did. She was an absolute game changer. She shared everything—her knowledge, what she'd learned from experience, her open heart. She taught me about abundance. Both corporate America and the yoga industry can be really competitive; her generosity was like a breath of fresh air.

But it came at a cost. Not from her but from the other teachers, who were territorial. They didn't understand why she'd come in from out of the blue and immediately taken such a big role when they had been there much longer. She and Anne instantly butted heads. Immediately, a competition ensued and they started jockeying for position.

Katrina had a rocky start. To smooth over some of the territorial vibes, I called a get-together at my house for all the teachers to meet her. She showed up an hour late. First impressions are a big deal, and that kind of thing is hard to recover from. From that experience, I learned a lot about how to communicate and make big changes with grace, mostly by learning firsthand what *not* to do. I should have communicated with the team way earlier and in person, before Katrina even came on board. I could have cleared the air, let people ask questions or express their concerns. I could have set the stage for Katrina to be successful. But now it was too little, too late.

In the meantime, Martin and I were apart. A few days after our breakup, he called to let me know that he'd hit rock bottom and was getting help. He *was* ready to deal with his demons. Ready to transform. He quit drinking and started running, meditating, praying, journaling, going to church, and seeing a therapist. These habits were all familiar to me. Now he was doing them too. Hallelujah. Since he was still not working, he spent his days immersed in working on his well-being. When he stopped drinking, he lost most of his friends. He started going to support groups to deal with some childhood trauma he had experienced, which I was just now learning about.

He also told me that his therapist said that she did not understand why I insisted that he go through this process alone. I had to work hard not to feel guilty about that. But I knew deep down that he shouldn't depend on me; I had learned that lesson in my own transformation. He needed to deal with his demons himself.

Over the next several months, he transformed. He became the person I'd fallen in love with. He was no longer numbing his pain from abuse and abandonment with alcohol. He rid himself of toxic relationships. To me, the most important thing was that he was doing it for himself. At first, I thought he was doing it to win me back. But when he kept going on his own, without my help, I knew it was for him.

During that time, I dated other people. I dated an attorney who loved yoga and Lululemon, and an older, wealthy real estate guy for a hot second. Though both were sweet and they were enjoyable experiences, it didn't take me long to understand why people say that the dating world is not as appealing as it might seem to those in long-term relationships. And my heart longed for Martin, especially around Christmas. I called him from Spokane, and it was clear that both of our hearts were broken and both of us were lonely. I yearned for the day we could be together again.

I started yoga teacher training with Katrina a few months later. I admit that I was doing the bare minimum at my accounting job, just trying to squeak by and nothing else. My plate, as usual, was overly full. My boss started to avoid me. My business partners were champing at the bit for me to buy them out. And I was training to be a yoga teacher. I could tell there was another big surge about to take place.

Rick and Tom had consolidated their efforts, and I could tell they were ready to make an exit . . . no matter what. They were distancing themselves, posturing for the buyout. They called a meeting with me in an office space they'd rented just for that purpose. Alone in a conference room, I sat across the big table from them. There was some intimidating body language going on, which I was accustomed to. In my job as an executive, I sat across from men like them all the time.

Tom and Rick laid out the plan: if I did not buy them out and give them what they wanted, they would sell the studio.

Sell the studio? They couldn't do that without a unanimous decision, per our operating agreement. Except that we'd never signed it. Previously, every time I brought that up, they made excuses to not finalize it—there were a few things they needed to look over first or they'd get to it next week when they had more time. Of course, next week never came. Not once, however, did I think they were intentionally bamboozling me.

They said that since there were no signatures on the agreement, majority ruled, and they could sell the studio if they chose to. They used scare tactics. Scare tactics require lying and provoking fear. Selling the studio would take a ton of time and money, which they did not have. I was about truth, so I did not even wince. I refused to be bullied. I looked them square in the eyes and said, "Sell it, then. Go ahead and try."

For them, this was not my typical response. For so long I'd been trying to prove myself to them, scrambling to please them and running at their beck and call, because I wanted them to like me, love me, see me. I did not need that anymore.

I got up, walked out of the room, got in my car, and drove away. I did not cry; I half smiled with my head held high. I was truth, I was me.

That conversation was a wake-up call, and after that night, I started getting serious about the buyout. I started to shop for a loan and quickly discovered that the bigger banks preferred to work with businesses that were at least three years in. We'd officially been running for only a little over a year. I wasn't sure how I was going to get financing.

Rick's girlfriend worked for Plaza Bank—a small bank that catered to minorities. She put me in touch with a loan officer, and I applied for a small-business loan. That was the first time I was even remotely considered for the loan. They had strict guidelines and a lot of hoops to jump through, but I was willing and ready.

I told my loan advisor, Max, my story. He was inspired by it and moved to help me. It also didn't hurt that I still had my accounting job, so I could personally guarantee the loan. I had a third-party valuation for the business done, and I did everything else I needed to do. The last step was to have a meeting with the president of the bank. Max told me, "Inspire him. Show him what you got."

So there I was, sitting at a large, black, marble table, across from two high-powered men . . . again. With confidence, I shared my story and my vision for the studio. I remember looking over at Max, who was wide-eyed and smiling, as if to say, *Yes! Nailed it!* That was the moment in which I saw the me that had been there all along. I got the loan.

During teacher training, I befriended one of the trainees who happened to be an attorney. He helped me draw up the purchase and sale agreement to present to my partners. Now I had the loan and the contract. I was ready to close the deal.

Then, while driving to the studio, I got a call from the bank.

"I'm sorry to have tell you this," Max said. "There's something wrong with the loan." My heart dropped into my stomach. He went on, "There's something going on with your credit that you'll have to address."

I knew exactly what he was referring to. I'd given the house to Eddie in the divorce, but my name was still on the mortgage because he could not refinance it on his own. Now, he was in arrears, which tainted my credit score.

It's going to be OK, I told myself. *No matter what, it will be OK. I have been through so much and survived. I will find another way.*

I parked my car, walked into the studio, and went behind the desk to check in the next class. And who should arrive but two avid students, Jeri and Amy. They stopped at the desk to chat.

"Hey," one of them said. "Do you ever think about opening another studio? If so, we would love to help." I was floored.

"Actually," I said, "now that you mention it, would you want to own part of this one?" They looked at each other, and I could see the excitement on their faces. A silver-platter gift from the universe.

I still worked to get the loan. After everything that had happened, I wanted to be the sole owner of the studio. Amy and Jeri were supportive and told me they would do whatever they could to help. They ended up floating me some money to make it happen.

In July 2011, I bought out my partners, became the sole owner of hauteyoga Queen Anne, and graduated from yoga teacher training.

Martin told me, back when he'd just started therapy, that every time he went for a run, he imagined that I would be at the top of the hill waiting for him. Now I was ready to be at the top of the hill for him. One day, after several months of being apart, when I knew he would be running at Lincoln Park, I went down there and waited at the top of the hill.

His surprise was priceless. He wrapped his arms around me. He knew. We were back on.

Over the next several months, I got accustomed to the next phase of my life. I was running the business on my own, without the constraints placed on me by my former partners. Tom and Rick took off to California. They'd washed their hands of me, though they believed I wouldn't be able to do it without them. It was strange to think that, just one year earlier, we'd been best friends, leaning on one another, making our dreams happen, getting through the hard times together. I did not think I would ever see them again. Another death, another rebirth.

In this new phase of our relationship, Martin and I no longer went out on the town but instead went running and played tennis and stayed in. It was different but the same.

I was more focused on the business than ever, and my work at Laird Norton suffered because of it. My heart just wasn't in it anymore. I started to make mistakes. I felt isolated and cast out.

And to top it off, I'd started teaching yoga, which, if you've never done it, I can tell you is an incredibly vulnerable space to be in. The team I built was very experienced. Most of them had five to fifteen years of teaching under their belts. Meanwhile, I had always been simply the owner of the studio. No one looked at me as a teacher. I had done everything backward. I was the only teacher I knew who owned a studio before teaching.

The only thing to do was jump into the deep end of the pool. I ignored my inner critic, who told me I was not ready. *This is my house,* I thought. I had put so much of my life into it, and now I had to trust that it would support me, hold me up. I just had to show up fully. There was no time to waste.

That first class, I looked around at the students. Every single one had kindness in their eyes. Teaching felt natural, here in the community I'd built. The familiarity created confidence in me. I was home.

Not to say that it was all smooth sailing from there on out. About one year in, I questioned myself. Was I good at teaching? Was I meant to do it? I still felt that people considered me the owner, that they weren't really looking to me as their teacher. I was attached to an idea of what a teacher was supposed to be, and I was comparing myself to the most experienced teachers. I had not fully found my voice.

One weekend, Martin and I drove up to Vancouver, BC, for a weekend getaway. On the way, I told him how I was feeling.

"Just be yourself," he said.

"But I still plan everything—every word, every pose, and every sequence. I basically write a script for each class! I'm afraid not to."

"Focus on your storytelling and let go of the script," he said.

I decided that day that I was going to stop trying so hard. I was going to let things be more organic, to speak from my heart. I decided to let go of my attachment to what the students thought of me and whether they considered me a teacher or a business owner. Both of those roles were important, and either way, it didn't matter. I got clear on what I wanted to bring to my classes: I wanted to inspire people. I had gone through so much to reveal myself, and I wanted to help others do the same. I was going to show up and allow myself to be fully seen.

After I became clear on that mission, I was a very good teacher, the teacher I wanted to be. I created a daily inspiration, a quote, mantra or personal story, and I started speaking from the heart. To this day, my classes revolve around that daily inspiration, using poses to *feel* it.

I was so grateful to Jeri and Amy for floating me the money for the buyout. Immediately afterward, they were still interested in opening another studio, and I told them that I would consider it. I was hesitant, though. I'd just gotten full ownership of hauteyoga and didn't know if I could do it again. But sometimes silver-platter gifts from the universe come when we might not feel ready for them. I couldn't turn away the gift just because I was uncertain and scared. I had to see where the opportunity might lead.

We started looking but took it slow. These ladies were selfless. They wanted to help people. I appreciated that so much. At the same time, they had an idea of what small-business ownership was but had never experienced it. I wanted them to see my life and exactly what it took to run a small business.

It did not take long before they saw just what the life of a small-business owner entailed. We mutually agreed not to enter into a partnership for a second studio, but instead, they would invest in the business. With their loan, I would build the second studio on my own.

Then, in October 2011, still working at my corporate job, a week after I filed all the corporate tax returns for the year, Ned, my boss, called me into his office.

"Please," he said, gesturing to a chair, "take a seat." He went and sat down behind his desk. He continued, his tone formal. "Leah, it is time for you to go. I will tell the staff that it was your decision, that you resigned."

I sat there, stunned.

"You'll need to leave the building at once. You can come back in a few days to get your things."

It took me a moment to collect myself. I nodded and stood up. Though leaving my accounting job was ultimately what I wanted, I always envisioned doing so on my own terms, exiting the building with two middle fingers in the air. I was robbed of that. I felt scared and helpless. That job was the last piece of the old me, of my old life, that I was still holding on to. It was also my security blanket, a six-figure income.

I was embarrassed and ashamed. I grieved the loss of my mentor, Ned, and felt bad that I had let him down. For years after, I told people that I'd left corporate America. I didn't divulge the whole truth. I didn't want people to see my failures.

Even so, it was the final death in my transformation. No longer was I compartmentalized into CPA Leah, Yoga Leah, Partner Leah, Friend Leah, Wife Leah. I was only one person, the same person in every sphere of my life. I was Leah.

Transform Cycle Reflection Questions:

1. Are the whispers of change and transformation becoming louder? What are those whispers?
2. Are there childhood traumas, dysfunctional relationships, or destructive behaviors you have been diverting or neglecting?
3. Was there an event in your life that caused you to look deeper within? Divorce, job change, loss, or death?
4. Are you stuck in a cycle, a repeated pattern that is blinding you from seeing opportunities for transformation?
5. What are you afraid of? Do you actually know those fears will come true?
6. Are you open to the signs and gifts from the universe guiding you to transformation?
7. Do you believe you have the courage, gumption, and strength to go through transformation? If not, why?

The Purpose Cycle

"What you are seeking is seeking you."

—*Rumi*

Once we've recognized and brought our disparate selves into a single whole, we can start to live our true purpose in life. But the work is far from done—to be honest, the hardest work is yet to come. In the Purpose Cycle, we find clarity. The true natures of our relationships are revealed. Honesty might lead to forgiveness and reconciliation, or it might lead to tightening boundaries or saying goodbye. We see people in a way we never have before, because we see ourselves. Love becomes greater. Pain becomes greater too. The willingness to feel everything stokes the life forces within us. This is where life really begins.

The year of 2012 was one of the best of my life. I was completely free. I was divorced, independently owned my business, and was out of corporate America. I spent that year hanging out with Martin, traveling, going to yoga festivals and retreats, enjoying the fruits of my labor at hauteyoga Queen Anne, and searching for a location for the second studio. I was surrounded by a community of yogis and new friends. I was learning, growing, and manifesting my life. It was a magical time.

Near the end of 2012, a commercial leasing office called to let me know that I could open my yoga studio in their space. It was in the exact area I wanted to be, an area that was growing but whose prospects were uncertain. My intuition (and practical analysis) told me to take the location. I would take on this venture alone. No partners, just me, myself, and I, risking it all.

I was afraid. While driving to Spokane with Martin for the holidays, I cried the whole way.

"I don't know if I can do it all again!" I said through my tears. "What if the new studio fails? What if I lose the stability I've worked so hard to achieve? If I fail, will I have to go back to being a CPA? What if I lose everything?"

I didn't really need to open another studio, I reasoned. hauteyoga Queen Anne was profitable. It was sustaining my lifestyle. The community I'd created was amazing. I didn't need more. But I knew I had a purpose, and that *this* was my purpose. I wanted to reach more people, to keep growing and evolving, to make a greater impact on the world.

I looked out the car window at the nothingness of the flat, snowy fields. The day was gray, the clouds low in the sky.

"Leah," Martin said. "You aren't growing if you're standing still."

There was no way to know if any of those fears would come to pass. Why do we fear what we do not know? Even if they did become reality, I knew I would be OK. I had failed before and survived, and I could do so again.

And so I decided to keep going. I knew I had to take the risk, do the work, and be brave enough to go after it, not only for myself but for the thousands of people who might be touched by my efforts. After the holidays, I signed the lease for the new space. Everything was about to change.

My strategy for building the second studio was a continuation of what I did with the first. I wanted a strong community that fostered creativity and authenticity. But it would be different than hauteyoga Queen Anne, with its own name, vibe, and culture.

The yoga industry had changed so much in the four years since I'd opened hauteyoga. Back then, there were only a few studios with hot yoga classes that offered creative movement and a soundtrack of mostly mainstream music. Fast-forward four years, and every neighborhood hosted one such studio. Some might have argued that Seattle was saturated with studios.

I chose not to take a competitive approach, instead holding to the idea of abundance. I believed there was enough for everyone and that a scarcity mindset was based in fear. I wanted the name to reflect that. Martin was the one who found the word *shefa*. It means abundance in Hebrew, healing and recovery in Arabic, and divine light and flow in a Spanish dialect. It was perfect.

I opened shefayoga Roosevelt in the Roosevelt neighborhood of Seattle on April 13, 2013.

In order to keep hauteyoga intact and create a new community, I kept the businesses separate and hired a whole new set of teachers. I was the only teacher at both studios. That was definitely not the easiest way to do it, let me tell you.

At the same time, I wanted the momentum from hauteyoga to reach shefayoga. It was naive to think that people would make the connection without an orchestrated effort on my part. People were busy and had other things on their minds. Which means I started from scratch.

For months almost no one showed up. I felt like my worst fears were coming true. Money was running out, and I had to take some of the cushion I'd built up at hauteyoga and invest it in shefayoga. There were times when I was not certain I would be able to make payroll or rent. I took out high-interest loans to make ends meet. I had a little more empathy for my former business partners, who had done the finances while I was running operations. Now I was doing it all and constantly felt the quake of financial panic.

Through it all, I did my best to remain steady. I got creative in driving business. I continued to nurture relationships with my teachers and students, meditated on mantras of abundance, and tried to remain present by taking one step toward the next step. I read that an elephant's gestation period is nearly two years, in which time a dog could have three litters. Big things take time.

I hired Martin as my marketing director (more on that later). We created brand videos and photos, hitting a fancy marketing campaign hard. While this certainly helped, what we were showing was not reality. We crafted the image that shefayoga was killing it, when it was really struggling.

This is the world of marketing and social media; this is how it works in business and in our personal lives. We put out images of happiness, success, and perfection even when we are struggling. There is a fine balance between wanting to promote happiness and joy in the world and just plain embellishment. But nothing is perfect, and one snapshot—or marketing campaign—is not the whole picture. Just as a disappointment isn't the end of the story, though it might feel that way at the time. It may be the beginning of a new adventure.

Katrina was still my teacher at this time, an incredibly creative person, a wise and articulate storyteller. When we first started working together, she was an inspiration to me. We had a lot in common. I was excited to learn from her. She's what I call mystical. I was never quite sure how all the stories she told lined up, nor was I sure where I stood with her.

As I mentioned, she had a rocky start with the other teachers. Katrina and Anne were engaged in a territorial battle from the get-go. I was determined to try to build a bridge between them, so we all could live in harmony. I did this because Anne was important to me, both as a friend and for my businesses. Katrina was also important to me. Over time, I started to see her not only as a mentor but also as a mother figure, whose attention I was still so desperately craving. In many ways, Katrina was like my mom: She kept me close but not close enough. I doubted that I could reach her or that I was secure. I always felt like she could leave at any moment.

There were countless times that I tried to douse the fire between Anne and Katrina. Both were convinced that the other was out to sabotage them. It was an ongoing drama that I got caught up in, trying to fix it so neither of them would leave, neither of them would abandon me. I was so attached. I thought I couldn't sustain my businesses without them, or that the studios would suffer significant damage if either of them left.

No matter how hard I tried—and I tried really, really hard—I could not get Katrina to see me. See me for who I was, see what I wanted her to be for me, see the love I had for her. I spent countless hours over several years sitting with her face to face in coffee shops, consoling her; writing emails to her to explain or justify my and others' actions; writing emails to my staff to explain or justify her actions; giving her opportunities;

building her up in public and in private. But no matter what I did, she always reverted back to "you love Anne more than you love me" language and behavior. I finally threw my hands in the air, threw in the towel. The situation was sucking my energy dry.

I learned that we are all blinded by our own wounds and not necessarily available to see someone else. I also recognized my attachment to her as a maternal figure, which was not healthy and could never give me the security I craved. I had to let go. I was so disappointed.

I decided that I was no longer going to have a working relationship with her. That meant she would not teach classes or trainings at either of my studios any longer. This would be a huge hit for my businesses. I decided I would create my own curriculum and lead my own teacher trainings. I was not sure I was ready for it or that I would be any good at teaching teachers, but I had to give it a try, start a new adventure.

Around the time I was about to let her go—I was waiting for us to wrap up teacher training at shefayoga—she seemed to check out. She just didn't show up to work or return calls or texts. I knew she was having personal issues, but she had always kept me at arm's length, so I didn't really know what was happening.

Then she left. No goodbye, no explanation. Someone whom I loved and had worked so hard to understand and support simply up and left. I grieved, crying for days and days. I was mad at myself for repeating the cycle of attaching to a mother figure who would abandon me. I was disappointed that I hadn't seen myself and had allowed myself to live in that chaos for as long as I did.

It is easy to do, to live in a repeating cycle that we are so caught up in that we can't see it. But it was from that experience that I became aware of my pattern, my habit of attaching to women in that way, and I vowed to see it faster next time.

That was one of the biggest lessons I learned in therapy. Our deep-seated issues, patterns, and triggers will never really go away. We just get better at identifying them and are able to get back to the truth, the light, quicker so we suffer less. Darkness is in all of us and is necessary for growth, but we don't have to live there.

Ultimately, Katrina and I never reconciled. I struggle with this, especially on my quest of reconciliation and forgiveness. But I realized, that's life. Sometimes, not everything can be fixed. Though I was disappointed in how our relationship ended, I will be forever grateful for all that she taught me. I also forgive her and myself for the suffering I endured.

After Katrina left, it was like a veil was lifted. I felt in a visceral way that nothing is permanent, that everything is fleeting and everything changes, and that grasping tightly and not letting go is futile. The only thing we can do is keep growing and learning from past mistakes. I've had plenty of practice because of all that I have lost and all that has changed.

Being in the business of people, I had to keep flexing my muscle of nonattachment and embracing change. Teachers and students moved on, most often because they had grown and were entering the next phases of their lives. Why would I ever want to hold them back? Why would I want to hold myself back from learning whatever their departures were meant to teach me?

During this time, my leadership style began to shift. Instead of focusing on what my teachers could do for me or how they could add value to my businesses, I started looking for the blind spots in myself, the ways in which I caused harm without knowing it. It's like driving a car. In order to see the blind spot, we have to do a head check. I was doing a lot of head checking. I studied how I interacted and reacted. I am a fiery, strong-willed person with an intensely compassionate heart. I have high expectations but give people many chances.

I lead with assertive love. I asked myself some tough questions. What was I doing that prevented growth? How could I be more approachable, more kind? What could I do to invest in my teachers so they would invest in me?

That effort to recognize my own impact—instead of putting blame or responsibility for how things were going on others—changed everything for me. I spent more time with my teachers. I began to really listen to them. I owned my shit if I failed to communicate well or handle an issue appropriately. I didn't do this to try to get them to stay forever, but to facilitate growth and expansion for myself and for them while they were there.

The relationships that I built are incredible. I have the most loyal and invested relationships with my teaching staff. Two of my teachers, Sean and Ginger, have been with me since the beginning, nearly a decade! All of my teachers call upon me, and I work to be there for them, to give them advice or just be a friend who can offer a hug and support. Now, even when they leave, I try to maintain a connection with them. So whether Casey decides to hike the Pacific Crest Trail for the next year, or Adrienne focuses on opening her own studio, or Puja flees to Washington, DC, to start a new life, or Anne tells me she's moving to San Francisco after being with me since day one, I don't crumble. Instead, I smile and wish them the best and tell them I am looking forward to our continued, though different, relationship. Because I practice nonattachment and embrace change, I suffer less. By suffering less, I can see more clearly and get closer to the truth. And that truth is love.

Right after Katrina left in 2015, I created my third business, a teacher training school called Sendatsu Evolution. *Sendatsu* means leader or guide in Japanese. I built a program that not only taught yoga poses and philosophy but also, based on my experiences, leadership skills and self-study. I was very careful in how I structured the curriculum, out of respect for Katrina. I strove to create something different than our other programs.

Not only do I love teaching people to become yoga teachers, I have found it to be an integral part of my purpose. I am only one person. If I can teach others to be leaders in the world, they will show others how to be leaders, and the ripple effect goes on and on and on.

While building Sendatsu Evolution's program, I was reading Brené Brown's *Daring Greatly*. That book had such a profound effect on me that I chose to include it in the program. The idea of courageous vulnerability became the backbone of my program and is what fuels so much of what I do today. Brown's vulnerability prayer was a huge inspiration for this book: "Give me the courage to show up and let myself be seen."

Back when Martin started working as the marketing director for both studios, I was a little nervous to mix business with our personal relationship. I was a lot nervous about the finances of hiring him as a salaried employee. I was naive in thinking that it would bring us closer.

As you might have guessed, our relationship became out of balance. We still lived apart, rationalizing the choice as both of us "wanting our space" and not wanting to deal with the logistics of living together. In reality, we did not see each other that much. He worked from home, and I was bouncing between studios and working at my house. But when we were together, we talked about work all the time, on date night or when we were at one of our homes making dinner. I was an organized businesswoman who wanted to know what was going on. I quickly learned (or relearned) that Martin did not like to be managed, and he did not want to be accountable to me all the time. With our equally strong personalities and desire for independence, we got into epic power struggles. Several times in a two-year period, I suggested he become an independent contractor, doing projects as needed, but he was adamant about having the stability of an employee. I tried to embrace this. I tried to release control.

It didn't work. Eventually, we started fighting a lot, and he started to retreat. I could not go through that again.

It came to a point where I suggested we go to therapy together. Martin and I had both gone to counseling individually, but we had never done couples therapy. Martin was game—we both knew we needed help figuring out how to manage our power struggles.

We got a therapist. He wasn't great. In fact, many times I caught him dozing off midsession. But he served as the holder of the space—he made us accountable to show up on a regular basis and do the work. Martin and I had been practicing honest and loving communication, so he didn't have too much to facilitate. Still, after several appointments, Martin began to abandon me, to go dark for days at a time. *How are we back to this?* I thought.

That was too much for me, and I decided to end it. Martin was argumentative and a tenacious negotiator, so I knew I would need help. I planned to do it in our next session.

When we showed up, I told Martin I needed to end the relationship. He was distraught. Emotional. Sobbing. He begged me to reconsider. I loved Martin. I wanted it to work. We had been through so much together. My heart was compassionate. The therapist suggested we try a "one more chance" solution.

"Can you put your issues on the shelf for one week and focus on why you love each other?" he asked. "That means no discussions about the things that are hurting you. Most people can't do it, but I think you should give it a try."

We did it! We hung up our issues and concentrated on love. We avoided talking about work and were intentional about showing our gratitude. We rekindled the light. From that day on, whenever our issues came up, Martin stayed in the fire with me. He did not retreat or abandon me. He stayed.

Over time, I was able to release the reins around work. I gave Martin full freedom, with little to no accountability to me. Let me be clear: this was not easy for me. I had to ward off feelings of being taken advantage of and a lack of gratitude, and I had to fully trust that he was doing what was best for the studios.

Financially, I carried the burden. I held up both of our lives. I made huge sacrifices. Eating out was usually on my dime. Travel was always on my dime. There were times I had to take out short-term loans to carry the businesses, which wouldn't have been necessary if I hadn't had to pay his salary.

I had numerous conversations with Martin over the years about this. I wanted him to get other contract gigs, which he did sporadically. I wanted him to notice my efforts more frequently and show more gratitude. But his pride often kept him from "making a big deal about it."

Taking care of everything—and then growing resentful about it—was a pattern for me, a cycle. I'd been the main provider in my marriage too. I still believed that without my oversight, everything would fall apart. It was a control thing:

When you manage it all, you control it all. If you control it all, they can't leave.

By this time, I had been exposed to many amazing teachers: Sean Corne, Sadie Nardini, Jennifer Pastiloff, and Meghan Currie, to name a few. They had a huge impact on me. I continued to hone my voice through storytelling and daily inspirations during class. I began to understand just how powerful words are.

They say that sticks and stones may break your bones, but names will never hurt you. I call bullshit on this. Words invoke dreams and fears. Words can create or destroy. Words can make or break us. They can mean the difference between life and death. I saw this in my classes. So many students left crying, energized, inspired, or simply different because of what I had said. I received cards, emails, and messages all the time confirming this.

One day, I happened to be standing at the desk at shefayoga when the phone rang. It was an avid student named Jax.

"Hey, Leah," he said. "I wasn't expecting you to pick up, but I am so glad you did." He went on to tell me that he was going to prison for a white-collar crime. He had been in litigation for a long time, and he was facing a twenty-year sentence. It was the hardest thing he'd ever been through, and he admitted that most days he wanted to take his life. But he kept coming to yoga to hear what I had to say. He told me my words saved his life. They inspired him to not give up.

I already knew I was fulfilling my purpose, my dharma, and that what I was doing was important. But his words relit the fire within me, the fire of deep commitment to my purpose. I knew I was making a difference. He helped me get clear on my intention and why I wanted to continue to teach.

———

I wrote in my journal later that day:

> Why I teach yoga:
>
> I don't do this because it is cool
>
> I don't do this because I want to nail a handstand
>
> I don't do this for the likes on Facebook or Instagram or any other external source of praise
>
> I don't do this for money, success, or power
>
> I do this to help people LIVE
>
> This is my promise! My prayer: God, please know this is my intention and help me live my purpose.

It is a big honor to be asked by the yoga clothing giant Lululemon to be a brand ambassador. Over the years, I had watched many of my fellow teachers get the honor. I waited and manifested—meaning I had a clear vision and hope, while taking action and letting go of the timing—that one day I would get it too.

Everything happens in perfect order. Right about the time shefayoga was stabilizing, I was asked to be an ambassador. It was great timing because I was out of the trenches of keeping my businesses afloat and now had the space to continue my own personal growth.

Being an ambassador is not about promoting Lululemon's clothing. It's Lululemon's way of giving back for their ambassadors' support and community building, of showing appreciation for their ambassadors' efforts and wanting to take a vested interest in their ambassadors' continued growth and expansion.

By now, being an inspiration through teaching and storytelling was the foundation of my work and who I was. I was even more dedicated and passionate about reaching people and helping them see their truest potential. I wanted people to break free from conformity and see themselves for who they really were, not what others wanted them to be. I was excited about all the people I could reach in the yoga room, but I wanted to reach even more. I wanted to inspire those who might never come to yoga.

At the first Lululemon ambassador meeting, we did an icebreaker. The facilitator asked, "If you could be a fruit, what fruit would you be?" Funny question, right? She answered first, to kick it off. She said, "I would be a pineapple. Pineapples come out looking the way they are, and they just get bigger. We are who we are; we are just waiting to show more of ourselves." I loved her answer.

The Lululemon team then asked me to write down my ten-year goal plan. They wanted me to visualize where I would be in ten years, then work backward to create actionable steps for getting there. This was the first time I had done goal setting like this. I felt vulnerable, and there were parts of me that did not want to proclaim some big, hairy, audacious goals. Lululemon calls these BHAGs. The voice of my inner critic was on a loudspeaker. But I told myself, *If I proclaim it, I will do it.*

I wrote down three big goals:

1. I own three yoga studios
2. I teach yoga retreats worldwide or own my own retreat center

Those first two weren't all that intimidating. They were business. I knew how to do that. The third goal was much harder to admit and commit to, and I hesitated before writing it down.

3.   I am an international inspirational speaker
      and/or an author

I remember thinking, *That is lofty and I have no idea how to get there, but I have to manifest it. I have to believe there is a way. I know I have the capacity to do it. If I am going to teach people to be as big as they can be and go after their purpose, I have to lead by example.*

It was easy to put that third goal off and focus on the other two. The journey continued.

Around that same time, Oprah came to town on her Live Your Best Life Tour. I got tickets for myself and Martin way up in the nosebleed section. I remember listening to all the inspirational speakers, waiting, hoping to be inspired. When we were on our lunch break, Martin asked what I thought of the program so far. For some reason that I didn't understand, I felt disappointed and frustrated. Later that night, after spending some time processing it, I realized I didn't belong in the bleachers. I wanted to be down there on stage. I continued to manifest and see my mission, my purpose.

Lululemon has thousands of ambassadors worldwide. A select few are chosen every year to attend their Ambassador Summit in Whistler, Canada. In 2015 I was chosen as the representative from Washington. There were around one hundred others invited from all over the world. This was a five-star event at the Four Seasons Resort that ran for four days. It was *epic*. There were various speakers, leadership break-out rooms, and tons of fun team-building exercises like scavenger hunts and dance competitions.

I was so excited. Being a leader could get lonely. Everyone was always looking to me for the answers. When something was broken, I fixed it. If there was a problem, I solved it. Most people wanted something from me, whether it be advice or a paycheck. I had been manifesting finding more peers, leaders who were doing the same things I was and didn't want or need anything from me.

But life is funny. I'd had some huge wins and things were looking up. My businesses were growing and so was I. It seems that, in those good times, the universe has a way of coming in and bestowing some perspective.

When I arrived at the summit, I found that I knew no one. Instead of camaraderie, I felt an air of competition. Everyone was on their A game. The voice of my inner critic came on a loudspeaker again, saying things like, *You are not good enough. Who are you to be here? Everyone here is better than you. You do not belong.* The voice was deafening. I did my best to quiet it and keep going.

Despite being intimidated and insecure, I managed to learn from many empowering and inspiring leadership exercises. I also made some amazing new friends—Regan from Utah, Jill from Oregon, and Audrey from Florida—whom I kept in touch with long after the summit. Audrey now teaches at hauteyoga!

The dharma talk focused on growth, and how, as we grow, we become more of who we already are. This theme kept repeating as a reminder. So often, we think we have to change. So often, we look outside ourselves to feel complete, worthy, deserving, or accepted. But everything is already within us. We just need to allow it to be revealed, to be seen.

At the summit, I learned a lot about utilizing my strengths. Just because we are good at something does not mean it's a strength. If we don't enjoy it while we are doing it but only enjoy its completion, it is not a strength. It is possible to love what we are doing *while* we are doing it.

That was a huge wake-up call for me. As a business owner and accountant, I still did everything, never asking for help because I thought I could do it better and faster than everyone else. I thought this was a strength, even though I'd begun to dread doing paperwork. I didn't want to do bank reconciliations anymore! With that realization, I decided to get a bookkeeper as soon as I got home. I would save my time and energy for the things that brought me joy and served the world.

The most eye-opening lesson for me was at the end of the summit, on the second-to-last day. In an exercise called Quieting the Inner Critic, about forty of us sat in a circle on the floor and wrote down something that our inner critic constantly said to us. The inner critic is that negative voice that tells each of us hurtful lies about ourselves. I wrote down:

Who are you to be here? You are not worthy.

Then we crumpled up the papers and threw them in the circle.

"OK," said the workshop facilitator. "Now, one at a time, each of you is going to pick up a piece of paper and read it aloud. Then the person who wrote it will come up and claim it." *Fuck!* You should have seen our faces.

The things people wrote blew my mind: "I am fat." "I am ugly." "I am not enough." "I am alone." "I am a failure." "I don't belong."

I was dumbfounded. As each person came up to claim their paper, I thought, *No! You are beautiful! You are enough!*

Why can we see this obvious truth when it comes to other people but have such a hard time seeing it in ourselves? All that time at the summit, I'd felt like I was alone, like I didn't measure up. And most importantly, that no one else felt the way I did. Then I discovered that *everyone* felt the way I did! As my paper was read, I got up, trembling, took my paper, and sat back down. I just sat there and cried. I could not believe how all these amazing people were up against themselves, just like me. We all have an inner critic. We all battle fear. We all want to be seen and to belong.

That exercise changed me forever. I only wish we'd done it the very first day. That would have leveled the playing field and allowed us to love and accept each other and cheer each other on sooner. We were told to "shake it off" as they played that song by Taylor Swift on the loudspeaker, and then we left to go to lunch.

Many retreated for the night. I think that exercise was really intense for some people, and they wanted to be alone to process it. I loved the exercise. The level of vulnerability it involved was off the charts, and people showed just how truly brave they were. This type of vulnerability and bravery needs to be nurtured.

I went to the facilitator later that night and told her my thoughts about doing that exercise sooner in the summit. She agreed and told me she would take my suggestion to the powers that be. I'm not sure she did, but regardless, I needed to speak up. Vulnerability is about having the hard conversations that reveal the truth. I vowed to use that exercise going forward.

A few months after the summit, Lululemon invited me to speak at what they called The Bonfire Sessions. They put together a series of events that involved different inspirational talks from leaders in various fields in our local community. I was honored that they asked me. It was my goal to reach people outside the yoga room—now I'd be getting my chance.

On a Wednesday night in October 2015, more than one hundred people gathered at Broadcast Coffee next to she-fayoga to listen to me speak for an hour and a half. I was used to speaking for small pockets of time in front of my classes, but having all eyes on me for that long was definitely new and nerve-racking. Many of my trainees, colleagues, family members, and friends were in the audience.

I shared my heart. I finally told the whole truth about being fired. Before this, I just said that I'd left corporate America, which wasn't exactly a lie, but I always left out the part about my being fired. It was the first time many of my friends and family heard the truth. I decided, on that night in front of one hundred people, I was going to own it, to show my humanity through vulnerability, and harness the courage it takes to be fully honest, fully seen. It was one of the most exhilarating and humbling nights of my life.

After it was over, I could not watch the video. The next morning, I woke up in a panic. *I have said too much*, I thought. I felt raw and naked. Brené Brown calls this the "vulnerability hangover." And let me tell you, it was fierce. I kept replaying in my mind what I had and hadn't said. My inner critic was yelling loudly.

Fortunately, that morning I had a personal training session with Dawni Rae. The moment I got there, she held the space for me—she attuned to me both emotionally and physically, giving me 100 percent of her attention. She literally held my feet and said a guided meditation to nourish me after I had given so much of myself. That kind of support meant a lot to me, and it helped me find my footing again. My inner critic started to quiet.

Back at the studio, I was able to receive the outpouring of love and support that came my way after the talk. I witnessed people owning some of their shame, and some of my teachers told me that they hadn't felt "ready" before but now wanted to work with me. In fact, one of them, Michelle, became my director of yoga a few years later. By allowing myself to be seen, I gave others the inspiration and permission to be seen.

After the Bonfire Session, the floodgates opened and opportunities to reach audiences outside the yoga room poured in. I was asked to write articles for businesses and do interviews for podcasts, videos, radio shows, and magazine articles. One of my students, Hylke, interviewed me for a book he was writing about leadership called *Taming Your Crocodiles*. He wrote an article based on my interview and got it published in the Harvard Business Review online and in the book *HBR Guide to Changing Your Career*! There was some irony to this: I'd been a CPA for fifteen years, but it wasn't accounting that got me recognition in the Harvard Business Review, it was being a yogi entrepreneur! Once we start taking action, no matter how scared or uncertain we are, the doors will open. We just have to walk through them.

I went on a vulnerability kick. I wanted to be fully transparent, to own all of who I was, all of my successes and my messy failures. I realized how much keeping the secret of being fired had been holding me down. I could not believe how freeing it was to just tell the truth and relinquish the shame. I committed myself to letting go of anything I was ashamed of and standing in my truth and light, to being and feeling fully seen.

And so I went shame hunting. I examined my life for areas about which I felt shame.

Earlier in the summer, after the leadership summit, I was lying on the grass at the lake with a few very special people in my life. As a rule, these people were unafraid to talk about politics, religion, women's issues, whatever sensitive topic ruled the day. We managed to maintain a refreshingly nonjudgmental environment.

Then the topic of abortion came up. I talked about what I "would" do, in the hypothetical. I did not fess up to the fact that I had been faced with this choice, and I'd chosen abortion.

One of them told us that he and his wife had given a baby up for adoption while in high school. They did not believe in abortion. As he shared this very private memory, I stayed quiet. He was so vulnerable and brave, and yet I recoiled. My reaction went against everything I was trying to be. I didn't own my truth.

Fast-forward to my shame-hunting quest. Here was a glaring ball of shame that I had to acknowledge. Up until that point, only Martin and I knew about the abortion. I'd rationalized for years that it wasn't anyone else's business. Which was true. At the same time, abortion is a medical procedure that many women undergo, and I believe that if more of us talked about it openly, we could diminish the stigma. And by talking about it, not only do we relinquish the shame around it for ourselves, but we allow others to release it, too, and together we are not alone. We are not bad. We are whole and good. Our bodies, our choice.

I didn't regret my choice. But I realized that not regretting it wasn't the same as not being ashamed of it. So I decided to write to my friend from the picnic. In telling him the truth, I was able to deal with the shame and grief I'd buried. His response was kind. He was proud of me for telling him the truth and told me that God forgave me. We have an even closer bond now than we did before. Vulnerability breeds connection. Martin and I started talking about the abortion, too, and he told me some of his feelings that I had never acknowledged. Together we felt the grief, and we allowed ourselves to cry and heal.

In 2016 I headed into the second round of Sendatsu Evolution teacher training. It's interesting to watch the students on the first day. They come in full of anxiety and fear, but by the end of the day, they understand that their fears are unwarranted, that they are strong and capable. To me, that is what self-study is all about. Yes, they will learn subject matter, but ultimately it's about pushing themselves outside of their comfort zones, about being vulnerable and brave. They have to dig deep within themselves to endure.

Nearly all Americans are required to be in school through twelfth grade; if they are lucky, some go on to college. Usually, formal education ends around the age of twenty-two. Perhaps this is why adults become stuck, fearful, numb, stressed. What if we were required to study our whole lives? The world would be a different place. There would be less fear and more openness, truth, mindfulness, and consciousness.

That is why I am committed to self-study, and I encourage all my students to be committed too. I study my behaviors, my past, other people, and my dreams.

Dreams are metaphors, stories from the subconscious that often don't make sense but do convey a message. My dreams are vivid, and one dream from that time period still sticks with me. In it, I'm running a race at the Olympics. I don't care about the medal; it's more about doing the best I can. I can feel myself crossing the finish line with ease and grace, then looking up at the ranking board and seeing that I won the silver medal. I can't believe it. I stand on the podium, crying, thinking I've defied all my limitations. After that, I return home and everyone is asleep. No one knows or cares, but I know, and that is all that matters. When I awoke, the messages were clear:

1. Do the work. Don't attach yourself to the result, just enjoy the process and do your absolute best, and you will do things you never thought possible.
2. Not all your work will be acknowledged, appreciated, or seen, but you will know in your heart what you have done.

3. Never stop growing, studying, or seeking. There is no
    final destination. (Which, I believe, is why I won the
    silver, not the gold!)

So there I am, headed into a new teacher training, knowing
that my own vulnerability is going to come up, and that I can
use it to model for and teach my students. I'd been a Lululemon
ambassador for two years, meaning I was coming to the end of
my term as an active ambassador. In my last goal-setting session, one of the facilitators wanted to know what I had accom-
plished and for me to reestablish where I was headed.

She said, "Leah, you can do this on your own. You have it
all figured out."

Actually, I did not have it all figured out. A pitfall of being
a leader is that people think I don't need any help, that I can
hold up the world. I needed support. I needed someone to hold
me accountable and push me out of my comfort zone.

"I need you," I said, a lump forming in my throat. "My pri-
orities have changed. Being a speaker has moved up the ranks."
I knew what her next question would be.

"How are you going to get there?" she said. I knew the
answer. It'd come to me a few months prior. An inner voice
had whispered, *Write a book. Call it* Seen.

Most speakers, leaders, and coaches have books as part of
their platforms, so I knew that's what I needed to take the next
step. Though I had heard that whisper, I had not told anyone
yet. Writing a book would be the ultimate gesture of vulnerability. Though I desperately wanted it and knew it was what I
needed to do, the thought of saying it out loud made me want
to throw up. I was so scared. My inner critic was on a loudspeaker again. *What will others think? Will your story be com-
pelling?* Everyone would find out about all my mistakes, my
failures, my humanness. I swallowed.

"I am going to write a book," I said.

Her response? "Of course you are! That is what we want from you. We don't go to your classes for the poses, we go to hear what you have to say!"

Gah! Holy shit. I am doing it.

I was buzzing. I went home, and the first thing my daughter said was, "Are you OK?"

"I just proclaimed something really big."

"Is it confidential?

"Not anymore," I said. "I am going to write a book." She was so excited.

"I want to help you!"

"Well, you are going to be in it. Will you be OK with me revealing a lot about your story?" Alexis thought about it for a minute.

"Fuck it, Mom. Do it."

To hear my fourteen-year-old say that with such conviction, at the risk of her own exposure, sealed the deal.

Right away, I got my intention straight. No matter the outcome of this process, I was going to write this book for myself. It would be part of my healing journey and growth. I had been through so much, and I wanted to process it on the page. So, regardless if this book took me anywhere, I knew it would be meaningful for me.

The next few days were a whirlwind. I kept butting up against my inner critic, but a cavalry of support had arrived. I told my teacher trainees, who were very encouraging.

Gail, one of my yoga students, best friends, and mentors, was a bestselling author. And in that moment, a silver-platter gift from the universe. I invited Gail to our favorite café, Bounty Kitchen. As I approached her, she smiled at me with her kind eyes. After we ordered avocado toast, we sat down, and she helped me get started. Before this project, I hadn't written much beyond journaling, so I had a lot to learn. She navigated me through the process.

Dawni Rae was also helpful. During a personal training session, I told her how my mom and stepdad sometimes called me Miss Perfect. Though I hated that label and knew it was not accurate, there was a part of me that believed I had to be the perfect person they saw. Dawni Rae had me write what I was feeling and create a mantra. I wrote:

> You are human. Let yourself be fully revealed. You are not what people think you are. You don't have to do everything. You don't have to be perfect. Not everything is strong and successful. You have failed. You have made mistakes. You had shame. You have wronged people. But in your quest to be seen, you must accept and forgive yourself in your own humanness. Mantra: I am gentle while courageous in my self-acceptance.

After the session, Dawni Rae had to leave. "Stay here as long you want," she said.

I kept crying, with fear, with relief. Then I looked up.

On the wall, the seam of two mirrors met directly across from me. In the slightly distorted reflection, the seam passed through the middle of my face. On the right side, light; on the left side, darkness. It was like looking into my own duality, accepting the light and darkness within myself. My crying escalated. Dawni Rae's cat came over, sat down next to me, and began to lick my arm, as if to say, *I love you. You are not alone.*

Later that day, my inner critic dropped in for a visit. *Your story is not unique,* it said. I remembered what Malala Yousafzai said: "I tell my story not because it is unique, but because it is not. It is the story of many girls." I can—all of us can—tell our stories.

Then I thought about how, a few weeks earlier, I was struggling with my staff and team of teachers. I was also missing some of the teachers who had moved away and feeling defeated in my efforts to build cohesion.

So I went to Karina's class. Karina taught at shefayoga. She and I were kindred spirits and aligned in our visions for teaching. She was hugely intuitive and inspiring. That night, her message about transparency really resonated with me. After class, instead of giving a polite answer when she asked how I was, I told her how I was really feeling. She looked shocked.

"I had no idea you felt that way. Why don't you start asking for more support from the teachers?" she said.

"They might not show up," I replied.

"But *maybe* they will," she refuted.

The image of me sitting on the steps of my classroom after kindergarten that first day, waiting for my mom to arrive, crossed my mind. *What if they don't show? But what if they do?*

A few days after my book proclamation, Martin told me he was taking me out. He was acting suspicious. He would not answer my questions about where we were going and seemed nervous, like he was hiding something.

"We need to stop by a friend's house first," he said when we got in the car.

I did not recognize the house. I had never been there before. I knocked on the door. It opened and there stood a handful of my teachers, waiting to greet me. They'd thrown a Leah Appreciation party, spearheaded by Karina! They showed up. Those who couldn't wrote me letters.

I couldn't believe my eyes. I started crying. Karina stepped forward and pulled me into a hug. "I see you," she said.

Even with all that love around me, I had a hard time receiving it. I told myself, *I don't need to lead. I deserve this.* And I started to let go.

After dinner, Karina had me lie down on the floor, surrounded by a bunch of pillows. The teachers laid their hands over me and said sweet, loving things. They massaged me, held me, and gave me gifts. I just cried. I could not stop crying. It was a surreal experience and something I will never forget. They made me feel more seen than I had ever felt in my life.

My daughter once told me that we cannot see our faces without a mirror. It is one of the few body parts we will never see with the naked eye. I love this. If we never had a mirror, then we would truly have to see ourselves from within.

To be living authentically, standing in your truth with transparency, intention, and purpose, is critical when it comes to parenting. As parents, we either break problematic familial cycles or we pass them on. If we can't see ourselves, then we cannot see others, especially our children.

I was determined to break the cycles of my childhood. I did everything I knew to make Alexis feel loved. I wanted her to have everything, to never feel abandoned or afraid. But when she was young, I was in the Conform Cycle, focused on the external. So I gave her things: lots of toys, lots of treats. I showed her love with stuff.

But no number of toys could make up for my facade of having it all. I was an unhappy person, and she could feel that.

Alexis went through a lot, like all children of divorced parents. While the separation was happening, she was confused and scared, yet she only ever asked me once to get back together with her dad. One time, right after I'd moved into my new apartment near the studio in Queen Anne, I found Alexis looking out the window.

"Alexis, honey?"

She turned around. "I thought you'd left me," she said. That broke my heart. She felt abandoned too. She didn't talk a lot about it or show her emotions much. She didn't like to cry. But there it was, this thing I'd done everything to shield her from.

I became more intentional about self-work with Alexis. Whenever she was upset, I would sit with her until she could let her guard down and tell me how she was feeling. I encouraged her to cry and to simply feel what she was feeling. I also told her how I felt and let her see me cry. I stopped focusing on giving her stuff and instead began to focus on being there for her in a real and loving way.

The more I saw myself, the more I saw her as her own unique person, not an extension of me. I was in awe of this human I'd made, honored to see her as the exquisite individual she was. I vowed to continue to be myself, live my truth, walk my walk, and talk my talk, and I hoped that would encourage her to do the same.

To my surprise, my relationship with Alexis was tight, right up to middle school. Alexis and I were communicating well, and she had not turned the corner as most teenagers do, from being their mom's best friend to hating her.

I loved being naked, and so did she. The moment she got to my place, she would strip down to her bra and underwear, something I knew she didn't feel free enough to do at her dad's house.

"Mom, am I fat?" she asked me one day. Oh, the dreaded question of a teenager.

"Alexis, you are beautiful. How you feel is way more important than the pounds on the scale. As long as you feel healthy, strong, and confident from the inside out, that's what matters," I replied.

We talked about sex, about how to put in a tampon, and so many other things I would have *never* talked to my mom about. I felt lucky.

Then, at the end of sixth grade, we were walking into the apartment when I noticed cuts on her arms. My heart sank. This was completely out of left field. *Why is my daughter cutting herself?* Pause. Breathe.

When I felt slightly calmer, I pointed to her arm. "What are those"? I asked. She pulled her arm in, hugged it to her belly.

"Nothing," she said. She dropped her backpack and went into the bathroom. I followed her in and leaned against the sink.

"I'm going to sit with you until you feel like talking," I said.

"I feel depressed sometimes," she said after a minute.

"Why cutting?"

"I don't know."

"Does cutting yourself take away the other pain?"

"Yes."

I looked away, then back at her.

"Mom, I'm not doing it anymore," she said.

"I believe you. You know I'm here whenever you want to talk, right?" She nodded. I leaned over and kissed her forehead. "I love you, sweetheart," I said.

I left the bathroom. I left the apartment. I walked down the block and bawled my eyes out.

Over the next few weeks, I watched my daughter carefully. Then, as I was pulling into my carport, the school counselor called.

"Alexis and I have been talking, and she told me that she's having a hard time with her dad."

Eddie and I parented differently. I knew he had body shamed her before, and that sometimes he badgered her. Alexis and I had previously discussed her coming to live with me full time, but she wanted to stay at her school with her friends. But if she was hurting herself because of stress at her dad's house, I'd have to take action.

The counselor and I spoke further.

"Will you talk with Eddie?" I asked. "If this comes from me, it will not be well received. He'll listen to you."

The next day, Eddie and Leah Number Two called. I assumed the counselor had called them, but I double-checked and the counselor told me that she had not spoken to them. I tried to put them off, but they said it was urgent.

Life works in crazy ways. I agreed to talk to Leah Number Two. She and I had a solid relationship. We didn't talk much, but we were good at handling things. She told me that she'd picked up Alexis's journal from the bedroom floor and it had fallen open. (That's how she said it went down . . . seems awfully convenient.) Leah Number Two read what was there.

Alexis wrote about being in love with her best girlfriend. While I intuitively already knew deep down, this information still hit me like a ton of bricks. *My daughter is a lesbian?* Maybe the cutting had something to do with that, with her feeling the need to keep it a secret, or perhaps with her feeling shame.

I rejoiced. Yes, I rejoiced, because I believed we'd identified the real source of her pain and we could now deal with it. I explained to Leah Number Two that the counselor had called and told me that Alexis had talked to her about how awful it was to live with her dad. We knew it would be hard for Eddie to hear. And I knew he would accept her and love her no matter her sexual orientation. But he would be crushed that she had thought otherwise.

That night, I walked into her bedroom and sat on the edge of her bed.

"Honey," I said gently. "Your stepmom found your journal . . . Are you gay? Is this what all this, the cutting, your dad, has been about?"

She looked at me. "It's OK, right?" I reached over and pulled her into a hug.

"Yes, of course, it's OK! I love you and accept you just as you are. It does not matter who you love. Love is love. I love you no matter what. And anyway, I already knew."

"You did?"

There were some signs along the way. There are always signs, we just have to pay attention and not see only what we want to see. Not that all straight girls act the same way or want the same things, but she had never done some of the classics, like playing house or talking about marriage or babies. More relevantly, she'd never had a crush on a boy. The smoking gun: her computer screen saver was a photo of a pretty girl.

"I did. I see you."

She smiled. I could feel the weight of the world release from her shoulders. I was glad that she would no longer have to carry this alone. That she would not go years hiding and pretending. That she would not have to go through the pain that so many of us did. She could be seen for who she truly was.

We called her dad and stepmom. They both told her that they loved and accepted her. Later, Alexis reported that the next few weeks at her dad's house were "awkward" because they didn't talk about it. But at my house, we talked about it every day. I asked her questions, wanting to know as much as I could.

From then on, we were best friends. She told me everything, from the time she first found her clitoris to her first drink of alcohol, her first experience with marijuana to masturbation. Every time she told me something like that, inside I was thinking, *Whoa! I cannot believe she just told me that!* Followed by pure delight. Once, she said that she should write a book about all the things we don't typically tell our moms but that she has. She educated me about all kinds of new things. She knew many kids at school with different orientations and genders. I learned so much from her. We can all learn from each other if we are open.

After coming out, Alexis began to thrive. She was passionate about film. She was an artist and a writer. She loved animals. She was crazy excited about travel. She was open. She was loyal. She was accepting.

The story did not end there. One day, at the end of her freshman year of high school, I picked my daughter up from school. As soon as she got in the car, she said, "Mom, I have to tell you something." Gulp.

"What is it?" I replied.

"I think I like a boy." We looked at each other and laughed. I was shocked. I had settled into being the parent of a gay child. Plot twist.

"Why not explore it?" I said. "You don't have to be anything but yourself right in this moment."

For the next few months, she told me all about this boy. She talked about being confused.

"I spent the last few years thinking I was a lesbian. This makes no sense!" she said. To her, boys were much more difficult to understand than girls. She was still attracted to girls too. I told her that when she eventually had sex she would know a lot more. Who knew? She could end up liking both. Until that time, I told her to explore all her feelings. I didn't care what she decided because it did not matter. I would accept and love her as she was.

Meanwhile, I was still searching for a resolution with my own mother. I wanted badly to forgive, to rectify, to have some sort of reconciliation with her. I was at the point where I could have lunch with her from time to time, and every so often, I would go by her house for about an hour. I came to a place where I felt safe in my boundaries. Seeing my mom didn't mitigate my soul-searching—I was still trying to heal the wounds of abandonment and neglect. I sought out different kinds of healing modalities, like yoga, meditation, and conversations with others who had mom issues. I recall a conversation with Meghan, one of my employees. We talked about reincarnation and how maybe we chose our parents for this life. Maybe I chose my mom so I could do the work I needed to do and help others do the same. Maybe my mom played her role so that I could be who I am today.

I felt more at peace about my relationship with my mom, though there were times that I cried out to be fully healed, to not be so broken or wounded on this primal, intimate level. To not feel so hurt by the one who was supposed to nurture me, love me, see me.

One day during meditation, I realized that this wound had made a scar on my heart. A scar that was not visible but felt, a reminder of all that I had been through and survived. This scar was not ugly; it was a beautiful blemish that reminded me that I was alive and had a story to tell others. With that realization, I created a mantra that showed the beauty of heartache in a positive light.

> My mess is my message
> My failures are my future
> My suffering is my story
> My insecurities are my inspiration

———

Sometimes, we take two steps forward and five steps back. A few days before Christmas 2016, I dropped my daughter off at her grandparents' house to spend the night. At around ten o'clock, I got a text from my daughter while I was teaching our late-night yoga class. It said, *Mom, I'm scared. They're drunk and I don't know what to do.*

My first thought was, *They must be out to dinner.* So I wrote, *Don't get in the car.*

Alexis replied, *We're at home.*

All of a sudden, I was hot with anger. Everything that I had tried to protect her from was now happening. Every fiber in me wanted to get in my car and drive like a bat out of hell to their house. Instead, I breathed. *I'm coming to get you,* I wrote.

Knowing my history, Alexis replied, *It's OK, Mom, you don't need to come. No drama, k?*

I paused, breathed, didn't react. I did not call my mom and give her a piece of my mind or send her a text with a lot of swear words and exclamation points. I replied, *OK, Alexis. Text me if you need me,* then put the phone away. I had to trust that she would be OK. The next morning, when I finally went to pick her up, I didn't say a word.

A few months later, my mom asked me out to dinner for my birthday. After what happened at Christmas, I wasn't sure why I wanted to go. I told myself I wanted someone to treat me, to take care of me. Perhaps I wanted to test myself and them. Or maybe there was still a part of me that yearned to have a "normal" family.

I found out that this birthday dinner was going to include me, Alexis, my mom, and my stepdad. I hadn't been out with both my mom and stepdad in eight years! And usually, my sister Holly went along too. Still, I was convinced that they would be on their best behavior after so many years.

Alexis and I walked out of the pouring rain into Tulio Ristorante, a swanky place in downtown Seattle. They were sitting at the bar. My stomach dropped. My mind separated from my body, and I started to rationalize. *They're just having one drink,* I thought. *It will be OK. Be cool. Just get through it.* At the same time, I wondered, *Is this their first drink? Will they have more?*

We sat down at our table, and right off the bat I noticed that their behavior was odd. It was probably just the alcohol, but I wasn't sure. Then, when Alexis told her we were going to Paris that summer, my mom literally wailed. "I want to go to Paris!" she cried, making a scene like a three-year-old having a tantrum. *Just get through it.*

Later, after her second glass of wine, she said, "I am so proud of Alexis. She is so creative. Such a beautiful artist!"

"I know, Mom," I said. "I'm proud of her too."

"Well," my mom went on, "she didn't get it from you; you aren't at all creative. Don't you wish you were creative?" I felt like I was talking to someone who'd known me years ago. She didn't know who I was now. I took a deep breath.

"Actually, I am creative. I create every day."

"I guess you're creative with numbers." What? I looked at her cross-eyed. Pause. Breathe. *I created three businesses,* I thought. *I created an amazing community. I'm writing a book!* But there was no point. She only saw me how she wanted to see me. It wasn't worth the battle. *Just get through it.*

By this time, she and Bob were on their third glass of wine. I was now on guard and ready to leave if drama ensued. Then came time for presents.

Alexis and I have birthdays a month apart, mine in February, hers in March. "It's a joint birthday for you and Alexis," my mom said. *Wait, what?* I thought. *Aren't we celebrating my birthday?* She began to shower Alexis with thoughtful gifts centered around her art and memories from when she was younger. She gave me a gift card. I was turning forty-three, but all of a sudden, I felt like I was eight years old again! My heart sank. *Just get through it.*

I managed to leave in one piece. Outside the restaurant, Alexis said, "That went well." She had no idea. After that dinner, I cried for four days. On my actual birthday, I cried for hours. How could I let that happen again? How could I let myself revert back to that powerless, rejected eight-year-old girl? Why didn't I turn around and walk out when I saw them at the bar? Fuck. I wanted so badly for things to be different, but they weren't. Nothing had changed.

I grieved for the loss of my hope of having a different kind of family. It felt like one more goodbye. I learned a big lesson, though. I don't have to just get through it anymore. I have a choice. I have a voice. I just need the courage to use it. This is my life now.

Karina and I were on the same page. We were both passionate about purpose, and we liked to bring a message and inspiration in our yoga teaching. We were committed to helping people find their voices, to be who they are by breaking down the barriers of what is holding them back. Karina pitched me a specific program designed for this kind of personal development. I wholeheartedly accepted the proposal and she and I co-created the program. Sendatsu Evolution Next Level Leadership was designed for yoga teachers who have gotten their two-hundred-hour yoga certification but want to take it to the next level. The program gave them the tools and the space to practice honing their voice. It involved deep work. We dug deep into vulnerability, worthiness, self-confidence, and leadership.

We were embarking on our second round of this program. We never knew who would show up for this deep work. We didn't know their traumas or stories. We accepted anyone who was ready to really do the work. We got folks from all walks of life, and sometimes my inner critic came out to play. *Am I qualified to do this work? I am not a certified therapist. Can I hold space for these humans who have endured so much?* The universe gave me a sign in the form of Mastin Kipp. I read his daily coaching blog, and he said, "God doesn't call the qualified, he qualifies the called." I didn't need a degree to help people—I was called to do it. That was my purpose.

In the program, we got intense resistance sometimes. This was not easy work. It was vulnerable, uncomfortable, and downright weird at times. Karina and I had to hold strong to break through. One student in particular gave us a run for our money. Mary came to one of my dharma talks, and she was so moved, she cried. She craved community and was looking hard to find it. So she signed up for the Next Level program.

I noticed that Mary hid behind a book whenever she was not fully engaged. But when she was engaged, there was a fierce creativity that burned in her. I could feel she was holding back in her life much of the time.

In the program, we did all kinds of crazy voice activities, not only to get the students out of their comfort zones, but also to hear their voices, their expressions and inflections. Mary resisted. When it came time for her to participate, she literally folded her arms and said, "No!" At first, Karina and I allowed this as her free expression. But then it got more and more challenging. For the last exercise, we had the trainees stand up and share how they felt standing in front of the room, how it felt in their bodies, then express their feelings through movement. Mary hesitantly stood up last, and only because I told her to go.

"I am fucking pissed and I hate this!" she ranted. "I don't play this way."

We were in a voice workshop, so that was like a big "fuck you." Karina was leading the exercise, so I wanted her to handle the situation, even though I felt compelled to say something. Karina did not challenge her. The energy of the room cowered. The feeling was familiar, like the suffocation of being put in a box, shut down. Karina had us take a break.

"Karina, I need to say something," I said to her in private. How could I let a voice training be silenced the first day? I could not. I had gotten really good at hard conversations. They make us vulnerable, but they draw out the truth. The truth then sets us free. "We are the leaders of the group, and we have to act as such."

We agreed that I would take over for a little bit. As I brought the group back together, I asked how Mary made us feel. Each person expressed their feelings in a loving and compassionate way. I think they understood her because they were probably feeling the same way. Mary kept saying that being quiet and bowing out was her authenticity. Though I knew that was her truth, I knew it was not THE truth. I tried drawing more out from her by holding the space for her to express herself, but she would not budge.

I felt completely defeated at the end of the day. I felt shamed.

The other trainees pulled me aside to express how grateful they were for my leadership, and for calling out that conversation. Though I knew I did the right thing, I left feeling unresolved. I still felt emotional and disappointed.

Back at home, I continued to try to make sense of Mary's actions. I finally figured out what it was all about. What she wanted was not aligned with her actions; it was incongruent. She wanted community and connection, love and trust, but then she closed herself off, stayed quiet, and hid. She called it her truth, but all I could see was fear. Could I help her through her fear?

No part of me wanted to go to training the next day. But I knew the best way to heal is to deal. To go back in, stand in the fire, face the music.

I walked in feeling drained and depleted, but I found the strength to endure. Karina was leading another powerful exercise in vulnerability. Mary participated. The students had to look into each other's eyes and repeat, "What I don't want you to see in me is . . . ," and then fill in the blank. Each person was so brave to stand with another and fully see their deepest fears.

The next day, I woke up feeling renewed. I realized I couldn't make a person see if they didn't want to see or were not ready to see. We have to meet people where they're at. All I could do was my best to lead, to coach, to challenge my students with fierce love and compassion. I needed to walk my truth. I needed to raise my voice and not be silent. I needed to keep showing up, acting with love, and seeing each person as I saw myself. I knew I would not always get it right, but I had to do my best. And perhaps at the end of our journey together, I could help them (and myself) grow one step further.

The funny thing was, when Mary came to my dharma talk, she asked me why I was so good at building community. I didn't have a really good answer in the moment. But through that experience, I found the answer: I am good at building community because I genuinely love all people. I want all people to feel seen and that they matter. I want them to feel connected. I lead from this place with complete truth and conviction. People want the truth. They are attracted to the truth. I am congruent, the same person everywhere. Whether I see you on the street or at the grocery store or in the yoga room, I am the same. I will remember your name. My actions and energy are grounded in my vision, and that is what makes people trust me and keep coming back. I will do this for you too. I will walk in the fire with you, stay with you, see you. I believe that we can find the common thread of our desire for love, and I hope that one day we'll all be able to see ourselves in each other, to see our sameness while also seeing our unique gifts and the purposes that we are here to share.

Life throws us curveballs but also gives us delightful sur-
prises. Natalie came to work for me at the front desk when
she was eighteen years old. She was a slight young woman,
wise beyond her years. She was a dedicated practitioner, taking
yoga classes every day, sometimes twice a day. She was pretty
quiet and kept mostly to herself. After several years, however,
something started to shift. She and I would talk a lot about
life and our dreams. I had those kinds of conversations with
all my front desk staff. I learned that Natalie wanted to leave
college and pursue a career in yoga. She loved it and felt like it
was helping her, and she wanted to help others. I inspired her
to follow her heart. She did it. She quit college and entered my
teacher training program.

That's when her appearance started to change. She gained
weight. It was then that I realized she'd been battling anorexia.
Finally, during the program, she opened up about it.

I was always curious about the root causes that trigger
self-destructive behavior. I asked her about her relationship
with her parents. She had amazingly supportive parents, she
told me, with no abuse or known trauma in her past. She'd
seen many therapists who hadn't been able to come up with an
explanation for why she was suffering. Eventually she found
the right one. This therapist encouraged her to look more
deeply into her past. She was able to learn more about herself and make some important connections between experiences in her history and the problematic thought processes and
behaviors that she'd carried into adulthood. One day, the therapist asked her a profound question: What was your mother's
pregnancy like? Natalie didn't know, so she asked her mother,
who told her that she'd been a twin and that her twin had died
in the womb. Her mother had given birth to both babies—one
dead, one living.

This was absolutely mind-blowing to me! This was likely the trauma that caused her detrimental behavior. She'd never known of this death to which she was so connected. When she learned this information, she was freed. She was able to grieve and make sense of her years of suffering. Sometimes, we have to search for a different answer. There is no one catchall for why we do what we do, but we have to be willing to look a little deeper for the answers to be revealed.

Natalie was in the midst of her transformation while she was in my teacher training. She still lacked confidence but was growing, working on releasing barriers and finding her voice. After she graduated, she took my advice and started teaching. After about a year, I saw her develop into a really good teacher. I considered hiring her for a teaching position at my studios, but I wasn't sure if she had truly found her voice. I wanted her to take my Next Level Leadership program, which she did. But right before it started, I took her class and was absolutely astounded by how much she had grown. Next Level took her even deeper.

Today she is strong and healthy. She glows. She's many students' favorite teacher. She has found her purpose. She is seen and she sees herself. I am so proud to have had a hand in that.

In my Transform Cycle, I lost many relationships, some voluntarily and some involuntarily. In the same fashion, I resurrected some relationships.

Once my sister Holly got sober, she became an important person in my life, one of my biggest supporters. She was the one who cared for me when I was a kid, and I was so glad she found her way back to me. Not only is she my sister, she is my friend. She's now my student, too, and she goes on all my yoga retreats. She never holds back in telling me how proud she is of me. She is my protector, and I am grateful that she navigated her way out of her darkness and into the light. She is a pillar in my life.

If it is meant for us, it will not pass us by. That's how I felt about Rebecca. Rebecca was my childhood friend and the wife of my ex-husband's best friend, with whom I'd lost touch after the divorce. She and I were kindred spirits, and I mourned the loss of our friendship. I knew that she and her husband didn't understand why I did what I did, but Rebecca had a quiet understanding of my struggles because she had them too.

Four years had passed since my divorce, when I opened shefayoga and got a message from Rebecca. She told me she worked nearby and asked if it would be OK if she practiced at my studio. I was elated. She came to class a few times, and one day she came in early. We stepped inside the yoga practice room to talk.

"I missed you so much," I said, with tears in my eyes.

"Me too, Leah," Rebecca said. "For years I didn't understand what had happened with you and Eddie. I was so confused."

"I can imagine."

"It actually brought up a lot in my marriage. I really examined my own happiness. Fortunately, we were able to move through it and are still happy together."

"I am so glad, Rebecca."

"Now I really see you, Leah, and I understand why you did what you did. I get it. I am so happy you found your purpose and are happy in your life."

Rebecca continues to be my yoga student. Not only that, but she's created her own line of yoga clothing for children. I love full-circle moments. That is closure.

Seven years after I'd last seen Rick and Tom, I heard a rumor that Rick was back in Seattle. I wasn't sure if I ever wanted to see

Rick or Tom again. My body tensed up just thinking about it, which told me that something was unresolved and that I needed to come back to love, to release that fear and anxiety in my body.

One day I was walking into the studio when I saw Rick standing outside the Starbucks next door, with his usual drip coffee in one hand. He was talking on his phone with earbuds in, gesticulating with his other hand in his gregarious way. A million thoughts ran through my head as I approached. *Will he acknowledge me or pretend not to see me? Should I say something? Should I turn around and go a different way? Will he be kind or unkind? Am I ready for this?*

As soon as he saw me, he got off the phone and came over to me. He gave me a hug. What a delightful surprise! We chatted for a brief moment, and he acted as if we were the same old friends we'd been before the buyout.

I was confused by the interaction and had to shake it off. I had mixed feeling about him being back.

A few months passed, then one day, Tom and Rick were standing in the doorway of hauteyoga. I went over to greet them, feeling a bit territorial. Before I could get outside, they walked in. They acted like it was old times. They asked questions about the studio as if they were still a part of it.

After they left, I felt a little unsettled. Insecure too. I'd never felt good enough around them, always trying to prove myself. Now, all these years later, those same thoughts and feelings resurfaced. *What do they think of me? How do I look? Do they approve of what I have done and who I am?* I saw this in myself right away and stayed with it, investigating my triggers in search of the truth.

During meditation, I focused on forgiveness and gratitude. I was grateful for what Rick and Tom had helped me start, and confident in the knowledge that I'd successfully run the business for the past seven years. I'd made hauteyoga into what it was. And at the same time, I honored their part in it.

The next time they came in, they stayed a while. The studio was closed, so it was just us three. I took this as an opportunity to put myself out there, to free myself of resentment and anything else I was holding on to. I looked at both of them.

"I am so grateful for you," I said. "I couldn't have done this without you. Though it ended poorly, I've moved on. And, just so you know, I'm writing a book and you are in it." They laughed.

"So are we going to get to fact-check it?" Rick asked. I smiled.

"This is my story and my truth. So . . . um, no."

After this, I was finally able to understand that they hadn't intentionally hurt me. That people generally mean well but occasionally act with fear. Now when I see Rick and Tom, we stop and chat, or exchange a friendly hello. Maybe a laugh about old times. I don't feel the need to be seen by them. I see myself. It is pure freedom.

One night in the spring of 2017, I dreamed of my old boss, Ned, who'd fired me from corporate America. I woke with an urgent sense of deep gratitude. Up until that point, I was grateful for him pushing me from the nest toward my purpose, at the same time being hurt by how he did it, by just cutting me off.

Ned had a good heart. I knew he probably carried guilt from how things ended—he'd always joked about his Catholic guilt. I wanted to set both of us free. I wanted him to know that I held no hate or resentment, just love and gratitude. So I decided to email him. I had seen through social media that his job had changed. I googled him, and sure enough, he had a new email address for his new job. At least, I hoped it was the right one. I had to try. Here is what I wrote:

Hi Ned,

I have been meaning to contact you [for] some time. I just want to tell you thank you. Thank you for being my mentor. Thank you for opening my eyes to the city and to a different way of life. Thank you for being a support during the start of my yoga business and the failing of my marriage. Thank you for all you taught me. And thank you for our once friendship.

I know that letting me go was probably not easy for you. I was hurt for a long time. I felt betrayed. But as I reflect on who I am and where I am now, I am so grateful that you pushed me from the nest so I could really fly. I don't know how long I would have stayed in the security of that job had you not let me go. It taught me a lot about myself. I am a thriving entrepreneur now and my life is SO different. I am who I am supposed to be, I am where I am supposed to be. I am living my purpose. You were such a big part of my life changing. So thank you.

With love and gratitude,
Leah

This was a moment in which I embraced uncertainty, went on faith, and wasn't attached to the outcome. I was acting with unconditional love. To my surprise, Ned responded within hours. He wrote:

Leah,
Thank you for the kind email. I have often thought about you and wondered how you were doing. It's great to know that you are thriving, I am very happy for you!

Where you are has more to do with you
than with me. You have always been someone
who sees something they want and goes for it.
Someone that is very action oriented . . . you get
things done. I also wish you the very best!
Take care,
Ned

What a sweet exchange. An exchange that happened because
I allowed myself to show up and be seen. I saw him, and he
saw me.

Holding on to the past only causes our own suffering, like
drinking poison and expecting the other person to die, as the
saying goes. But if we allow ourselves to see the parts of us that
contribute to pain and suffering, and truly try to find awareness, forgiveness, closure, and understanding, this is where the
suffering ends. When we experience this and feel the lightness
and peace this hard work creates, we will seek to see more. It is
no longer about the other person, it is about us.

For a long time, I studied and practiced vulnerability. My
vulnerability muscle was getting strong. Like craving the
endorphins we get from working out, I craved the feeling of
vulnerability. I started to *seek* vulnerability. If I was not putting
myself out there, if I was not vulnerable, I was not growing.

I loved Olympus Spa, a women-only Korean spa. There,
women of all ages, sizes, colors, with one boob, two boobs, or
no boobs, walked freely in their exposed skin. The best part
was we all wore little caps. Without hair, we were all the same,
just different. I noticed that we all have the same parts, but we
are unique in small, precious ways.

There are stories written on the containers of our physical bodies that show where we have been. When I see all the
diversity in the world, I am reminded that there is no perfection. It is actually the imperfections and differences that make
us beautiful. When we are able to witness others being seen,
we realize that we are all enough. We don't need to be so hard
on ourselves. We can love the skin we are in and embrace the
uniqueness within our sameness.

Another way I seek out vulnerability is through different
healing modalities. I love sound baths, sweat lodges, Reiki,
energy work, and somatic experiencing. Somatic experiencing involves training the nervous system. Our sympathetic
nervous system controls our fight-or-flight response, which
turns on when we are under stress. Our nervous system does
not know the difference between being chased by a bear and
worrying over how many likes we get on our Instagram posts.
We are in a state of stress far too frequently, which puts the
sympathetic nervous system in overdrive. When we stress, we
suffer. We need to slow that down.

Andy, a healer in the Seattle community, reached out to
offer me a session of somatic experiencing. I didn't know him,
but he had heard of me and my businesses and wanted to practice on me, knowing I would likely be a good candidate for this
modality. Being open to new experiences and healing meth-
ods, I gave it a shot. After the first free session, I continued on
for several more. My sessions were literally me sitting in front
of Andy, the facilitator, looking at him or around the room.
There was not a lot of talking. This modality trains us to be
calm and present. It is a very vulnerable and uncomfortable
experience, and the client has to be open to the nothingness.
Wow, have I had some breakthrough experiences!

My very first session I spent staring at a birch tree outside the window. The tree reminded me of the birch tree that
was in the front yard of my childhood home. Andy asked me

about the tree, which led me to memories of my dad cutting it down. I was sad because I'd felt like the tree provided protection. Then I had a vivid memory of my dad holding me in a rocking chair, my body fully intertwined in his. I felt the pure, present, unconditional love of that moment. *He* was my protection. I started crying. I wished I could find this feeling with my mom. I had recently watched a movie called *Heart of a Dog*. It was profound. In it, the narrator says that if your relationship with your mother is strained, look for *one* moment of pure, unconditional love. I searched but could not find it, not even one. That day, I found it with my dad, and that was enough.

In another session, I felt antsy. I am used to being the leader, so it takes me a bit to settle in and let others take the lead, to just be. My feeling of anxiety was extra high that day, and it reminded me of the way I felt when I had this one recurring dream. I told Andy that in this dream I had at least once a week, I'm in some faraway place and cannot get home. I've just missed my plane or lost track of time.

"Why do you need to get home? Is something or someone in danger?" Andy asked.

I paused, thinking, then said, "No. No one is in danger. Everything will be OK if I don't make it home."

"Well, why don't you just stay, then?"

This blew my mind. Giving myself permission to stay, that I was OK no matter where I was. Wherever we go, there we are. Just stay. Everything was going to be OK.

Being a yogi, I was exposed to many spiritual practices. I experienced my first sweat lodge on a retreat in Mexico, then another in Venice Beach, California. A sweat lodge involves being packed into a small, pitch-dark outdoor dome with as many crouching bodies as can fit, to sweat for two or three hours. The ceiling is low and the floor is dirt, with hot coals in the center of the dome. It is quite a vulnerable situation.

For my first sweat lodge, I rallied the retreaters whom I was co-leading to try it with me. As soon as the door shut, my body responded by panicking. I wasn't expecting that. I rooted my hands in the dirt, breathed, and repeated, "I am here, I am here, I am here," over and over until my panic subsided and my breath and body came back to neutral.

For both sweat lodge experiences, there was a focus on drawing in our ancestors to recognize the path they forged for us. It's easy to forget about past generations when we get caught up in our nuclear family drama. By focusing on my paternal grandmother and grandfather, I was able to see how much I was like them, without any of the baggage I had from my mother and father. As I sweat, I saw the image of my paternal grandfather, who was a renowned doctor, holding out his hand as he was about to die, and I realized I was from him. I, too, had become a healer in a different form, and I was carrying on his legacy. The image of my grandmother was even stronger. She was a nurse and pioneer in mental health. She created Spokane Mental Health, and the organization named the building after her after she passed. I felt her presence. I felt her in the lodge, holding my hand, looking me in the eye as if to say, *I have paved the way for you, dear Leah. Keep my legacy alive. You are from me, live through me.*

There are so many souls who came before us and have been a part of our journey. There was so much growth, struggle, and suffering to sculpt the new grooves of our own existence. If we recognize this, we summon gratitude for what they bestowed on us. The sweat lodges helped me to feel loved and see myself within the honor of my lineage.

Another thing I like to do to seek vulnerability is get outside my comfort zone. One day, I decided to go on a hike at Pinnacle Lake. I initially wanted others to go with me, but my heart kept saying, *Go alone.* So I listened.

As I drove into the mountains, the GPS took me off-road for about six miles. I was not used to that kind of driving. Usually, I went on hikes where the road getting there was well paved and there was a parking lot at the base. Now, I was going less than ten miles per hour through giant potholes, without cell service or another human in sight. I started to get nervous, but I continued.

Eventually I made it to the trailhead. I was still anxious, thinking, *What if I get hurt or lost? No one will be able to find me.* I continued. The hike was steep, the trail full of raised tree roots. About a mile in, I came to my first roadblock, in the form of giant logs. The trail was not obvious; I looked for signs but there were none, so I followed my gut, climbed over the logs, and found the trail. I continued.

Then I came to the second roadblock. It became clear to me that I had gotten off the trail and was lost. I'd reached a dead end. I tried to find my way back to the trail and ended up in the brush. I thought, *You have to go back. You are lost. You don't know the way.*

Finally, after a fair amount of panic and some clumsy bush-whacking, log-jumping, and unsuccessful attempts to find my way, I got back to the trail. I stopped and breathed. Then, like magic, I saw the way. I was supposed to have gone left, not forward.

A sweet little lake, with the reflection of the mountains over it and little yellow flowers surrounding it, came into view. I sat down on a sun-warmed rock to rest. The stillness was palpable. I noticed there was more trail, so I got up, stretched, then continued.

Pinnacle Lake was a huge, pristine lake, with mountains and endless blue sky as its backdrop. I had it all to myself. It was magical. I stripped off my clothes and dove right in! Freedom. It was just me and a very persistent horsefly all alone in the crystal-clear water.

I was confident leaving. I knew the way.

When we seek vulnerability, we see that fear and courage intersect and that we are more than we thought. We see beyond the fears, move into the truth, and open up to infinite possibilities. We stop seeing what we aren't and start seeing what we are. We've just got to be willing to feel and then to see.

Part of my purpose is to serve, to be of service. When we make it to this last cycle, the Purpose Cycle, and go through the courageous transformation that needs to take place, giving back feels not only desirable but necessary. When we can serve from the place of our purpose, real change can happen because of our passion. I want to serve in order to help every person be seen. I have chosen to serve not only my own yoga communities, but also other organizations that align with my mission. Yoga Behind Bars is one of those organizations. It is a nonprofit that sends yoga teachers to teach in prisons. Prisons exist to literally hide people away, never to be seen again. But people in prison deserve to be seen and loved the same as everyone else. They are people who've been hurt and then hurt others. The worst thing we can do is not see them. In my journey of self-love, I learned to see each person as me. I have overwhelming love for prisoners, perfect strangers, and those closest to me, because I love myself. In order to love others, we have to be willing to see ourselves, because if we don't, we will never see anyone else, even those who need it most. We have to love each person as we love ourselves. I believe the way to heal is through rehabilitation, and yoga is one way to do that.

Everything happens for a reason. I do believe that. Some of the lessons are bigger than others. Some are so big they shake you awake.

In May 2017, hauteyoga became infested with rats in the ceiling. Seattle is notorious for its rat problem, but in eight years of being in the space, this was the first time they'd gotten in.

I was quick to respond. I called pest control, and after a few days, the rats were gone, or so I thought. Then, a week later, I got a call from the front desk saying that there was a rank odor permeating the yoga room.

I rushed to the studio. It smelled like death. I called the rodent specialist, who arrived quickly but could not find the culprit. It was like a disease without a cure.

"We'll come back tomorrow," the specialist said.

The next day, as I was driving in to continue to deal with the "disease," I got a call from the doctor.

"I'm sorry to tell you this," she said, "but your mammogram from a few days ago has come back abnormal."

Cancer. Disease. Death. The words rang in my head. I literally felt infested.

"You'll have to get more pictures done so we can see what's going on," the doctor continued.

Remarkably, I got to the studio without crashing. I couldn't do anything about the disease in my breast at the moment, but I could direct all that anxiety toward trying to cure the rat "disease." I admit I went a little crazy, masking the smell with incense and drilling holes in the walls to search. Nothing. I felt like I had no control over my studio or my body. All I could do was wait.

Later that week, I went in for more pictures. Martin took me because we needed to take his car to the shop. He dropped me off. I didn't know if he'd left or if he'd parked and come up to the office.

After, the nurse came to give me the results. She said, "Do you have someone with you?" Suddenly, it got scary.

"Do I *need* someone with me?" I asked. I frantically called Martin. "I need you in the exam room, stat." Fortunately, he was in the waiting room. He made his way back. Once he was settled, the doctor arrived. She said, "We've determined that you have two suspicious masses in your right breast. We'll need to do a biopsy." Gulp.

The two weeks leading up to the biopsy were a storm of internal struggle and emotional and physical pain. Just holding myself together required all my energy. I had to bring in all my tools for this one: being present, not attaching to the outcome, trusting the process. We were at the end of the Next Level program, and since I was teaching truth, authenticity, voice, and vulnerability, I decided to lead by example. I shared my story. As Brené Brown says, "Vulnerability is the catalyst for courage, compassion and connection." And it was just that.

Before the procedure, Martin told me he was going to North Carolina to visit his family and would not be there for it. I felt neglected and ungrounded. I made arrangements to have my sister Holly, Dawni Rae, and Karina there with me. It was still hard for me to ask for help sometimes, but I told myself, *I am worthy of support. I am worth being seen, even in my worst moments.*

The day Martin left, I took Alexis out to practice driving. It was her first time driving outside a parking lot. If you're a parent of a teenager, you know just how nerve-racking that first time can be. We were a block away from home, going down a hill with a sharp turn to go under a tunnel.

"Turn," I said. "Alexis, turn. Brake!"

She did turn, only not exactly in the same way as the road did. Suddenly, we were high-centered on a cement block, the car literally dangling. We managed to get out and down unscathed, but the car wasn't so lucky. Fluid was leaking everywhere. Martin was gone. I was supposed to teach in the next hour, then lead the often-emotional graduation for my

Next Level trainees, then get a biopsy the next day. They say God only gives us what we can handle, but this was pushing it.

I called the tow truck, got a substitute for my class, and made it to the graduation. It took every last ounce of me, but I knew it was my job to love and serve even in the midst of this crisis.

I had texted Martin right after the accident, and he responded with one text asking if we were OK, then went silent. I couldn't reach him, and my mind started creating stories. I went to bed feeling rattled and raw.

The next morning, I fully expected to see a message from Martin on my phone. Nothing. I began to cry uncontrollably. En route to my biopsy, I received a text from him saying that he was glad we were OK. I replied, letting him know how distraught I was about not hearing from him. No response.

The biopsy was traumatizing. I had to lie still, facedown, with my right breast in a hole cut out in the table, while the doctors and nurses pulled on it, took pictures, gave injections, and inserted markers for mapping the masses. The music playing reminded me of a death scene in a movie. Tears flowed out of my eyes and onto the brittle paper on the hospital bed as I breathed, meditated, and focused on a mantra and positive thoughts. The body and the mind react how they need to, and I did my best to let go of control. The nurse was so kind. She lightly patted my back during the whole process. Though it made me cry more, I appreciated her compassion.

After ninety minutes, I was allowed to get off the table. My body shook, and I felt weak, scared, and in pain. The nurse gave me some juice, and I pulled myself together before going out to meet my posse of amazing women. Holly, Dawni Rae, and Karina held me, cared for me, stayed with me.

Martin never called or texted. He was simply nowhere to be found. That torment was almost worse than the biopsy. He arrived back from his trip late the next night and came to my house and got in my bed. I was so hurt and angry. I pretended I was asleep. The next morning I was still distraught, and we got into one of those awful crying fights.

"Where were you when I needed you?" I sobbed.

"I decided to go to New Orleans to get some footage for the video project I'm working on," he explained.

"You couldn't even text me?"

"I was on my way back. I was on standby and then transitioning planes. I didn't have time."

"It takes two seconds to send a text. I don't get it!"

"I'm sorry, Leah. I just couldn't contact you."

"I don't understand this, Martin. I can forgive you, but I don't understand."

I had so many questions. Did I have cancer? If so, how bad? Could I die? Should I tell my daughter? Over the next two days, I had to sit with uncertainty, trying to ward off worst-case scenarios. The pain in my body and the bandages on my breast were a constant reminder.

I also had to come to terms with Martin's abandoning me. Was he getting back at me because earlier that year I had led a yoga retreat in Mexico while he had knee surgery? I racked my brain for answers and rationalizations. They didn't come.

I learned that I have to ask for what I want. It is one of the highest forms of vulnerability. When he'd asked me if I wanted him to not go to North Carolina, I should have told him to stay, or at least to be back before the biopsy. But I didn't want to put him out or be a burden. Even though I told myself that I was worthy of support, I was still learning to receive it. So many of us are afraid to ask for help or what we want, and then we're disappointed when we don't get it.

I decided to tell Alexis what was happening. Though I wanted to protect her, I also wanted to be honest. She was a strong young woman, and I trusted that she could handle the uncertainty. Plus, I had a feeling that she was going to be there when I got the results, and I needed her to be prepared.

When I told her they'd found something on my mammogram, she gasped. I will never forget her face. I explained the situation. She got quiet. I urged her to talk to me. She said, "Just let me feel what I need to feel right now." Touché.

The next morning, by chance (or not), Alexis had a late start time for school. Normally, she would be at school at seven, and I would be sitting in Starbucks working. Instead, she was home with me when I got the call at eight.

"Hello," said the nurse. "I called you first thing to let you know your results are *benign! Namaste.*"

I interpret namaste to mean that the light in me sees and honors the light in you. I bawled. Praise God. My daughter, hearing me cry, came and stood nervously in the frame of my bedroom door.

"I'm OK," I said, reaching toward her. She smiled, then came over and gave me a hug.

On the entire thirty-minute ride to school, my daughter held my hand. I was glad I had told her and that she got to experience one of life's inevitable curveballs by my side. She saw my vulnerability and celebrated with me. If we truly want to know our children, we must allow ourselves to be known by them.

That experience deepened my empathy for other women. The majority of students who practice at my studios are women, and many of them face hardship every day. We are all going through something, no matter how we seem on the outside. Kindness and love are what help us endure.

The only family member I told about the biopsy was Holly. Once I got the results, I decided to share the news publicly. I shared the lessons that I had learned during the process on Facebook, hoping to bring awareness and cause for celebration, not drama. It was also a source of inspiration for many of my yoga classes. Most of my friends and family cheered. No one took my wanting to keep it private personally. Well, except for one person: my mom.

That same week, I got a voicemail from my mom, in which she expressed how disappointed she was that I hadn't told her about my cancer scare earlier and that she had to find out about it with everyone else on Facebook.

I had been seeking resolution with my mother for so long. The breast cancer scare shook me awake. I talked it over with Martin and Dawni Rae, and they encouraged me to get clear on exactly what I wanted. Did I want an apology? Did I want more time with my mom? What did I want really?

What I wanted was for my mom to stop drinking. Not just when I was around but all the time. I knew if she really stopped drinking, she would have to do some serious self-work. I wanted to get to know her. The real her. And I wouldn't be able to do that unless she was sober.

The afternoon I decided to make the call, I sat in my car, staring at the phone. Telling myself, *I am the queen of hard conversations. Just call.*

It was a Wednesday at noon. I dialed, not expecting her to answer because usually she was at work at that time. I think I subconsciously did not want her to be there. By chance (or not), she picked up. She was alone, without my stepdad to march in and save her. I am pretty sure she was sober (it was noon, after all).

She went right into asking about the biopsy. I gave her the short version, but then told her that that was not why I'd called.

"I'm sorry you were hurt that I didn't tell you, Mom," I said. "But I'm also perplexed as to why you thought that I would. We haven't had a solid relationship for eight years. I don't trust you." She was silent. Stunned.

Her usual excuse to herself and others was that I was "too busy" to see or talk to her. It was time to dismantle that lie. I began to speak.

"One of the biggest lessons I learned from this experience is that I need to ask for what I want. It's time for me to tell you what I want, so that we have a chance of mending our relationship going forward. The reason I don't come around or communicate with you is not because I am too busy to see you. I make time for people I love and trust. It's because I don't feel safe with you. In order for me to feel safer with you, you'd need to get sober and stay sober for at least one year. This is what I want. Please do not contact me until you've been at least one year sober." Gulp. I had never straight-up asked her for this. It felt like a huge request. *Do I deserve to have someone change their whole life to be in a relationship with me? Yes, yes, I do.*

"I see your posts on social media about unconditional love. So how can you put this condition on our relationship?"

"This is a boundary, not a condition or barrier. It's not about unconditional love. It's about me feeling safe."

"Don't you ever have a cocktail or glass of wine? Don't you hang out with other people who drink, or can no one drink around you?"

At that point, I knew she was not ready or willing. There was a brief moment when I thought, *Oh, no. She is going to reject and abandon me.* But then it passed, leaving in its place a feeling of peace. I was not attached to her decision. She wasn't done, however.

"But we have been so good about not drinking around you! Isn't that enough?"

"Remember my birthday?" I said calmly. "That was an absolute disaster, and I felt terrible for a long time after. Holly and her husband say the same thing happens with them. I'm sick of this cycle, Mom, and I want it to change."

I had no expectations, but I had to ask.

Finally, my mom said, "I like my wine, but I will try. And I hope you know that I will always love you."

To me, this felt like a no, like a final goodbye. I wasn't sad, though. I felt liberated, completely free, with no ambiguity. My mom knew what I wanted—the ball was in her court.

After I hung up, I called my sister Holly and told her the story. She said, "Holy shit! You just did a phone intervention!" That wasn't my intention, but I could see how it would look that way to a recovering alcoholic.

"She's probably not going to change," I said.

"But what if she does?" Holly replied.

All I could do was try to manifest healing for my mother while at the same time completely letting go.

After I set myself free from that attachment, I had another significant shift. This shift was in my relationship with Martin.

Martin and I had been pretty complacent since our last stint in therapy. We were still not living together; he was working for me and doing side jobs sporadically. We had fallen into a routine, like many couples do. Still, I loved him very much and was fully committed to him. He was my person. We had been together for almost nine years (including the brief breakup).

I'd resisted living with Martin, not because I wanted my own space—that was just an excuse—but because of my deep-seated fear of abandonment. Now that I'd let go of some of that fear by setting a boundary with my mom, I felt brave enough to move forward with Martin. I was ready. Ready to break the routine. Ready to move forward. Ready for a fully committed partnership. Ready to ask for what I wanted. I was no longer afraid.

The way in which I approached Martin was not the most loving. It was more in the vein of a frustrated ultimatum. Note: That is not an effective way to ask someone to come toward you, let alone live with you.

I had grown tired of our back-and-forth, and I was a bit stunned that I had not seen it earlier. But big changes tend to happen one at a time and with growing momentum, like a snowball rolling down a hill. First we have to deal with the small things, which lead to bigger things, which lead to the REALLY big things.

Long story short, it did not go over well. Martin did not like being told what to do. Though I didn't approach it in the best fashion, I still couldn't understand his response. For him, it came down to logistics. Again. Who would move in with whom? Where would we live? How would we manage to live *and* work together?

"Do you really want to be accountable to each other one hundred percent of the time?" he asked.

"Yes," I said, "I do. I want to be in a committed relationship."

"Well, I don't want to be accountable one hundred percent of the time."

I couldn't help but hear my therapist's voice saying years ago, *Martin is not a relationship person. He will not be able to fully commit to you.* Though his reaction caused me concern, I still was not ready to see.

"I'm not asking you to move in tomorrow," I said, changing tactics. "I just want to take steps in that direction." He didn't want to sell his condo. The condo association allowed only a certain number of condos to be rented at a time, so the first step would be for him to put his name on the waiting list. He hesitantly agreed to do so.

"It could take years, Leah," he said.

"Well, at least it's a start."

Honestly, I didn't believe he would do it.

Over the next few months, I saw our relationship in a new light. It was like a veil had been lifted, but only halfway. I could see how out of balance things were, and try as I might, I couldn't get my head around him not wanting to be accountable to me. I kept pressing into that. What did that mean? I figured it was because he worked for me, and he did not want me to micromanage him at home too. Intuitively, I knew there was more to it than that. But I didn't yet have the courage to face it. I decided that I would ask him to find a new job because that would take the accountability piece off the table. He could still work for me on a regular basis, but I wanted him to start earning more of his income elsewhere.

I waited for the right time to bring it up. I knew he would resist, because I had actually tried several times before. He always talked me out of it. Usually, I brought it up during times of financial pressure, and he would simply say that things would get better. I would then refocus on my belief in abundance, that I could do it all, that the universe would provide.

This time, however, I was in the middle of doing the deep observation and contemplation required to write this book. I looked back at my journals. So many of the entries were questions about Martin's commitment to me and my resentment about holding it all together. Then the veil lifted even more. My go-to dysfunction was overfunction, which I worked to conquer by practicing delegation, trusting, and letting go. I'd succeeded in all areas of my life. All but one: my relationship with Martin.

He was always a huge advocate of my mission to let go of control. He'd say to me, "Just because you can doesn't mean you should." Except, of course, when it came to him.

I realized that I'd done it in my marriage, and I was doing it again. I hadn't taken the time to break the cycle. I still took care of everything. Car repairs, I paid. Vacations, I paid. New car, I co-signed. Salary, I paid. I had taken on many high-interest loans to keep my boyfriend on the payroll and my businesses afloat. Forget about saving money or finding a better home for myself and my daughter.

All of a sudden, I could see it so clearly, and what is seen cannot be unseen. I had to break the cycle. Now it wasn't about moving in together. The issue was much bigger. One that could not be negotiated or rationalized away. I had to stop: stop overfunctioning, stop controlling, stop holding it all together. I deserved to be supported emotionally, physically, spiritually, *and* financially.

Awareness is the first step, then comes action.

I truly loved Martin and wanted to be with him. I'd been so scared of losing it all. And because of that, I'd hindered our growth, both individually and as a couple. It had to end now.

For days I contemplated how to tell Martin. I wanted him to feel loving kindness. I knew it was going to be scary for him. I would be breaking a cycle that directly affected him and his livelihood. I was going to ask him to fend for himself. I knew he could do it, that he could rise to the occasion like he had before. *If he supports my journey, he will understand,* I thought. I hoped that asking him to find a new job would spur a breakthrough in our relationship, but I also knew that it could be the beginning of the end. Either way, it had to be done.

On a Saturday in early September 2017, the day before I planned to tell Martin, I was listening to a conversation between Oprah and Brené Brown. Oprah said, "In order to live a brave life, you are going to disappoint people, and those that truly love you will be OK with the disappointment and will accept your truth." I took that to heart. If he truly loved me, he would understand.

Sunday finally arrived. I was waiting in my apartment, pacing back and forth. As soon as Martin walked in, he knew something was up.

"Let's sit," I said as I guided him to the brown leather sofa in my living room.

"I love you."

He looked at me, perplexed. "OK . . ."

"And I need you to get another job."

He didn't say anything.

"You know how I tend to micromanage—"

"Yes, I'm aware," he said, smiling.

"I don't want to do that anymore. I've realized I need to make some changes. I am so grateful for the work you've done for me all these years. I want you to stay on as my marketing director, but instead of a salary, I will pay you as a contractor. This is fair and the way I've always wanted it." I paused, took a breath, then continued. "And I also need you to contribute to our relationship. Financially, I mean."

How we process loss is a strange phenomenon. At first, Martin was calm.

"Great, I want that too. How are we going to do that? I've been waiting my turn to build my career. You're going to help me, right?"

He felt my apprehension. I wanted *him* to do it. Then he started to deny and rationalize.

"I have done so much for your businesses. I've put you first, myself second, for your vision. I don't feel like you see that."

"I am truly grateful for all you have done for me," I said. "It was never my intention for you to put my vision before yours."

"OK, I'll do it. It will take me some time, but I will do it."

"I want the change to happen in the next four months, by the end of the year."

That's when he got angry. Anger equals fear. He went silent and retreated to bed. Neither of us slept well that night. Both of us tossed and turned, pretending not to notice that the other was awake.

In the morning, Martin wanted to talk about it. He told me that he felt misunderstood and unseen.

"I put my dreams on hold to help you build yours. I thought it would be my turn someday," he reiterated, like I didn't hear it the first time.

I had to work very hard to stand my ground. "I didn't make you do anything. I certainly didn't want to keep you from building your dreams. Working for me was your choice. I'll grant you that we were very focused on building shefayoga those first two years. But the past three years? There was plenty of space for your own growth. I can own the parts of this that are mine, and I hope that, once the fear settles, you will see your part in it too."

He collapsed in tears. I leaned in to him, wanting him to feel my empathy, compassion, and love. He tenderly received it. We stood together like that for a while, trying to stay in that peaceful, loving place.

The next day, I felt guilty. How could I cause so much fear and suffering? Was I being selfish? I reminded myself that living my purpose, my truth, was not selfish. It was an act of love. Being honest about my needs and living from my deepest desires was how I could serve the world the most. I saw that Martin was in pain, and I told him that this was an act of love. Love to myself, and ultimately an epic gesture of love for him. Not only would it prevent me from building the kind of resentment that would eventually kill our relationship, it would give him a chance to look at himself and grow.

As the days went on, we continued to talk about and hone our desires. He made it clear that he did not want to go back to corporate America. He wanted to have the flexible lifestyle he was used to and did not want to go "backward" into that life. I continued to communicate my desire for financial support outside my businesses. I didn't need him to get another full-time job. It could be anything: a contract job in his field, or a miscellaneous part-time job somewhere. That would be a step in the right direction. And who knew? That could be the start of him building his dream, whatever that was. "Growth will come from this," I assured him. "It always does."

That was one of the most interesting times I've ever had in an intimate relationship. To lean in and show up in full love and support, with no defense, only clarity of purpose, all while watching my partner flail, suffer, and struggle. To be fearless in asking questions or sitting in the silence of uncertainty and standing my ground. It felt mature, clear, honest, and loving. It showed that we could embrace our duality and the duality in our relationship, churning together, both of our hearts open. Instead of running, hiding, or retreating into the blindness of our fears, we were leaning into love. We were there together, fully visible, fully seen. Or so I thought.

The next few months were incredibly hard. Martin was in a fear-based place most of the time. Our relationship halted in many ways. We stopped going out and stopped having sex. He was barely eating or sleeping. I was having a hard time, too, but did what I could to allow him to ride the waves of fear and give support the best I could. "I'm in survival mode," he kept telling me, something I didn't understand. To me, survival means being willing to do anything to survive. Yet any ideas I gave him, he batted away. "I've tried that," he'd say, or:

"I looked there."

"That won't work."

"The commute is too long."

"It won't pay enough."

He was still looking to me constantly for answers and help. I had to be mindful of the difference between being supportive and falling back into a managing role again.

He eventually started to find gigs that interested him and seemed promising in some ways, but they weren't even close in terms of supplying the financial support I needed. But progress takes time, and I stayed in a place of positivity for him. He seemed to start to shift, too, and make his way toward me again.

Meanwhile, my work life was very full. I was leading teacher training and creating new events on top of running the two studios. Karina invited me to be a guest teacher on her yoga retreat in Sayulita. Sayulita was my spirit home. It was my favorite place in the world. It brought me such joy and healing. My initial reaction was, *No way, I have no time to do that right now.* But my heart and intuition said, *See if it could happen.* I told her it was highly unlikely, but I would look at my calendar. I checked and discovered I could actually do it! There were a million reasons for talking myself out of going, but everything in me said, *Go.*

The night before I left, Martin and I had sex for the first time in months. I was glad to be leaving on a high note and hopeful about coming back refreshed to find more progress on his side.

Instead of going to the lively and vibrant part of Sayulita, where I'd hosted yoga retreats nine times, we stayed at a retreat center called Haramara. It was quiet there; it was the place I was supposed to be.

One day after my arrival, I got a text from Martin saying that his computer had been hacked, that someone had taken all his information and now they were after him. Strange. He then called me, frantic, saying that they got my information, too, and were going after me and my businesses. What? He was using words like con artist, crazy person, and blackmail.

"Her name is Hayden," he said. "Do not engage."

Hayden called hauteyoga that night and left her name and phone number for me to call her back. I was so confused. A con artist or blackmailer would not leave me her full name and phone number. Something was not adding up.

I called Martin the next morning to try to get answers. He told me she was an old client with whom he'd done a photo shoot a while ago for really cheap. I kept asking, "What does she want from you? Did you take something from her and now she's trying to get you back?"

"I don't know," he said over and over. "She's crazy!"

"You need to call the police. I'm surprised you haven't already."

"I will," he said. "I'll protect you. Don't worry, I'll take care of everything."

I trusted him.

The next morning, I woke up in a panic. My curiosity and skepticism were overwhelming. I decided to google this Hayden person. I discovered that she owned a small business on Vashon Island. I realized there must be more to the story, and that this had to be a matter of the heart. I let myself sit with that for the day.

Meanwhile, on retreat, I was doing deep energy work (with *chakras*, for those who know yoga speak). I was standing strong in my power, having deep conversations with Karina about worthiness, and the understanding that what anyone does to me has nothing to do with me. I was full of conviction. I was glowing yellow in my third chakra (another yoga thing). I was preparing myself for what was to come.

The next morning, I walked to the open-air yoga *shala*, a place of practice and study. The shala sat high above the jungle and ocean. It had breathtaking views of nature. It was empty except for the ornate Buddha heads and mantles of intention decorating the space. I sat with my legs hanging over the edge of the practice room floor, over an abyss of trees, looking into the lush jungle of green and listening to the ocean waves crashing behind me in the distance below.

I took a breath and called Martin. I told him I was having trust issues and that what was happening did not make sense. I started to pull out the truth bit by bit. After much prodding, he finally told me that this woman really liked him, and he liked her attention.

"But I see her as a mentor, that's all," he said. Funny that he'd never mentioned her before. He went on, "She gives me good ideas and has taken an interest in me." Casually, he said that she was the one who'd given him the idea to go to New Orleans to shoot footage for a video project. "I like the attention, OK? Maybe she hopes that it will turn into something more, I don't know."

Finally, confirmation that this was indeed a matter of the heart and not some con artist going after me and my businesses.

That night, I talked things over with Karina.

"What if Martin was with her in New Orleans?" I said. The thought sickened me. I'd been so devastated when he hadn't contacted me during my biopsy. I'd never understood why he didn't even send a text during that time. If he was down there with her, whether for business or personal reasons, it would break my heart.

"Don't go too far down the path of assumptions," Karina said. Then we kind of chuckled, because it was somewhat of a preposterous thought.

The morning of my departure, it snowed in Seattle. It was only November third, so this was highly unusual. Martin was going to pick me up from the airport, and I had so many questions and a ton of dread. He was so good at talking me into and out of things. When I got to the airport in Mexico, I learned that my flight was canceled. They gave me the option to fly to Los Angeles and then Seattle the next morning. That was no coincidence.

I had four hours to kill before my flight to LA. I plopped myself down on the cold floor of the airport next to a phone charger and called Martin. I figured I might as well get some answers. He picked up, and I could tell just from the way he said hello that he was scared. I went straight to my burning question.

"Were you in New Orleans with Hayden?"

He paused. "No."

I was not convinced. "Were you in New Orleans with her?" I asked again.

Pause. "No."

"If I find out otherwise, our relationship is over for good. So I will ask one more time." This time, I rephrased the question. "Was she down there the same time you were?"

Pause. "Yes. But listen! She was down there with other business partners. We saw each other just once." He kept saying, "I did nothing wrong. I did nothing wrong!"

I hung up the phone and wept. In that moment, I did not care if it was personal or just business—his absence on that occasion was so traumatic for me, and now it was even worse.

He kept calling and texting, begging for me to pick up. I finally called back, and over the next three hours he tried to talk his way out of it. I kept reaching inside to see if I could overcome this. Could I forgive him? One thing was for certain: I did not have all the information necessary to make the decision.

I caught my flight to LA and stopped communicating with Martin, though he kept attempting to reach me. I booked the hotel nearest to the airport. It was after midnight when I arrived. Walking into the fancy lobby, I could hear laughter and sense the liveliness of the other guests. I felt far from that. I felt heavy. I checked in and went up to my room, dropped my bags on the floor, and kicked off my shoes as I looked in the mirror. My tear-stained face looked tired.

Dawni Rae called me.

"Martin showed up at my door," she said. "He's freaking out. He told me this big long story, something about a woman named Hayden being just a mentor and she's crazy and they're in some kind of *Fatal Attraction* thing."

"Do you believe him?" I asked.

"He was pretty convincing. I don't know; it seems like it wasn't anything more than some weird emotional relationship gone wrong. I really don't think he cheated on you, at least not physically. He knows he fucked up. He looks really bad, and he smelled like he hasn't showered in days. He hid under his hoodie the entire time we were talking. He kept saying, 'I don't want to lose my family.'"

"I don't know what to think. I don't know if we can overcome this," I said. I flew home the next morning.

At home, I showered and prepared myself to go to the studio to teach. Alexis happened to show up right before I left, saying she'd received a voicemail from Martin.

"It's like a goodbye voicemail or something," she said.

"Can I listen?" I asked. She nodded.

"I can't even listen to it all," she said. I took the phone from her and listened to the message. She was right—Martin told her to follow her dreams and be who she is. He did not sound good. I was upset at that violation.

Somehow, I managed to collect myself long enough to teach my class. During it, Martin left a text and a voicemail that seemed odd, in that same vein of a goodbye. I called Dawni Rae to see if she had heard from him. She, too, had received weird goodbye-type messages. That was when I started to get scared.

I drove home and told Alexis that I was afraid for him, and that I needed to go make sure he was OK. I had briefed Alexis earlier on what was going on between us, so she knew we were in crisis. I jumped in my car and headed for his place. Dawni Rae stayed on the phone with me the whole time. I was wailing in fear and frustration, angry that he'd pulled me in to take care of him once again. It felt like a desperate and manipulative move, but still my heart went out to him. I had never felt fear like that. I was petrified of what I was going to find. No matter how much pain he was causing me, I loved him and did not want him to die.

I parked the car and hurried into his condo, screaming his name. I found him on the bed with a bottle of whiskey and a bottle of pills next to him. I started pounding on his chest, screaming. He responded but just barely. *He's alive*, I thought.

"How much have you taken?" I shouted. He didn't say anything. I called 911. "Martin, you need to stay awake. Why the fuck did you do this?" I did not understand. I hadn't broken up with him; no decisions had been made. We were just navigating the situation, so why would he try to end his life?

Later, after the ambulance took him to the hospital, I found out that Martin had been very drunk but did not have a lethal amount of Oxycodone in him. Martin was released that night. I was so angry. His suicide attempt was almost worse than the situation with Hayden. How could he have done this to the people he loved? How could I trust him ever again?

The next morning, I had to teach at a big venue: Chihuly Garden and Glass at Seattle Center under the Space Needle. I was still showing up in my life, because that is what I did. Audrey, a teacher and friend, came to the event. I'd given her my house key so she could hang out at my place while I was in Mexico. When I saw her, I asked her if she'd stayed at my house at all. Her response stunned me.

"I went several times, actually, but every time I went, someone was there."

"What? Who?"

"There was a black car in your driveway and the lights were on. I didn't want to intrude, so I never went in. Someone was definitely there, though, I just didn't see who." It couldn't have been Martin—he never went to my apartment uninvited or without permission. Was it him? I was still scared that there was a crazy woman after me. Was it her?

Martin continued to send me texts, voicemails, and emails full of apologizes and proclamations of love. He promised to be everything he had not been. He begged and pleaded for me to give him another chance. It didn't make any difference, because I still didn't have the entire truth. I only knew parts. The parts he was willing to give me.

It was time to find out the whole truth. I'd saved Hayden's phone number. It was time to call her.

She picked up after a few rings.

"Hayden? This is Leah," I said tentatively. "I believe you tried to reach me a few days ago."

"Yes, Leah, hi," she said. "I'm not trying to cause any harm, but I think you should know what's going on.

"I agree. Will you tell me? I'd like to know everything."

I could hear her taking a deep breath. "Martin and I have been in relationship for a year and a half, since May of 2016. We met at a gas station. We went on a few dates, and it was mostly sexual in nature at first."

That was really hard to hear. Sex had been a point of contention in my and Martin's relationship. I was always asking for more, but he was always either too tired, sick, or his body was sore. It was a huge blow to my heart and ego to find out that he was giving it to another woman.

She went on, and I knew she was telling the truth the moment she said that they spent Wednesdays, Fridays, and Saturdays together. Those were the days I was with my daughter. So when I was with Alexis, he was with her, with Hayden. She said she liked that schedule because she was busy running her businesses and being a mom to her two kids.

She and I were living these parallel lives, which made it easy for Martin to live a double life.

She went on. "Martin told me that you were an ex-girlfriend but he still worked for you, and that he had a good relationship with your daughter. He and I dated casually for a while, then he began telling me he loved me a few months later, in December. We agreed to be monogamous at the beginning of 2017, in February."

That was when he had knee surgery. I was running a yoga retreat in Mexico at the time and could not be there, for which Martin made me feel terrible. "Were you . . . were you there after his surgery?" I asked.

"I stayed with him for the first three days after, yes. He needed someone to take care of him."

I realized that we'd both been sleeping in Martin's bed for a year and a half. We'd shared the same pillow. I felt like I was going to throw up. "He came to stay with me when I got home from Mexico," I said. "What did he say to you about that?"

"He told me that he wanted to be at the house of a friend who was a nurse and could change his dressings. He also said that he'd be staying in the basement, where there was no cell phone service, so he couldn't be in contact as much."

Finally, I mustered up the courage to ask the question that had been torturing me.

"Did you go to New Orleans with him, in May of 2017?"

"We went for our one-year anniversary."

What a blow. The breath left my body.

Finally, the truth.

That was not all. She told me that, a few months later, they went to New York for the US Open. To me, he'd said that he was going with one of his tennis buddies. He was completely integrated with her friends and family. She lived across the Puget Sound, only a twenty-minute ferry ride to a whole new life.

"I have a question. What big client did he lose?" Hayden asked me.

"That big client was me," I said. "I asked him to get another job, thinking that would bring us closer."

"I see," she said. "That's when he started to pull away from me. In fact, he ghosted me. I was angry and confused, so I went looking. I don't go on social media much, and I had no reason not to trust him. The answers were right there the whole time! I saw a photo of the two of you in Paris that summer of 2017.

He'd told me that trip was for a photo shoot for a coffee company. But you'd written something like 'my love' with a photo."

I bought that trip for him for Christmas.

"Well, after that I couldn't deny the writing on the wall," she continued. "I got pissed and told him that he better tell you, or I'd show you some of the emails he'd sent me."

"He told me that you were a crazy bipolar person after his identity."

For a moment, she didn't say anything. "My ex-husband is bipolar," she finally said. "Martin knew how hard that's been for me."

"That's awful," I said.

"Anyway, he still wouldn't come clean. He just kept on telling me that you and he had broken up for good in February of 2017, and that you just so happened to be in Paris at the same time."

"How convenient."

"Then I got some emails from you. They were really strange and actually sounded like Martin."

Aha! Martin must have been in my place when I was in Mexico, using my computer to send Hayden emails. He was the hacker! She promised to forward the emails she'd received from my Gmail address to me once we hung up. Later that day, they arrived in my inbox. Here's one of them:

> From: Leah Zaccaria
> Date: October 30, 2017 at 9:10:28 PM PDT
> To: Hayden
> Subject: I'm Done
>
>
> Hi Hayden,
> Martin and I have had a non-romantic relationship
> since February. He's good to my kid! Please leave
> us out of your relationship!

And that was that. The magnitude of the lies and betrayal was overwhelming. My first reaction was, surprisingly, gratitude. I was grateful for finally getting the truth. Had I not started to shake up our relationship, this could have gone on for years. So much more could have been lost.

My second reaction was sorrow for him. How could he have been that unhappy, or felt that unworthy, that he could sabotage something so good? I also felt relief for him that he no longer had to carry those lies. How exhausting!

My third reaction was utter disbelief. How could this have gone on for so long without one slipup? His absence during the biopsy had been a hint, but never did I think it was this. At least I was able to intuit that something was not right in our relationship and that I had to shift it.

We were broken beyond repair. Trust smashed to smithereens, and no coming back from it. I felt sucker punched. Up until that point, I was lobbying in my mind for how we could work it out. The truth shattered all my rationalizations. I kept saying, "This is not my life." And I think that was the exact message from the universe. This was not my life; this was everything I did *not* stand for. I taught and lived the truth, and I was sleeping next to a lie.

I assumed that Martin and Hayden were no longer in communication. While finalizing plans to meet up with Martin, I texted her to ask her not to tell him we'd spoken. She apologized and said she had spoken to him that morning. I was an hour too late. He knew I knew the truth. She forwarded me the correspondence between them.

From: Martin
On Nov 7, 2017, at 6:58 AM
To: Hayden
Subject: What happened

Please know that I'm very sorry for hurting you and for this whole situation. I know I don't have a right to ask, but I'm begging for your forgiveness. This situation is very tenuous. You could help me by not getting involved, and letting things try to heal. There's nothing you can do. There are a lot of raw feelings right now. I don't know what your first instinct will be. Please take a little time. Will you consider what I'm asking?

Please know how sorry I am!

From: Hayden
On Nov 7, 2017, at 8:11 AM
To: Martin
Subject: Re: What happened

Martin,

I believe that there is a part of you that is honorable, genuine and trustworthy. Please dig deep to live and love from that place.

Leah and I had a heartfelt conversation yesterday, and more lies were revealed on both sides. Feelings are indeed raw and your actions will have an impact on all involved for a long time.

Your request that I "not get involved and just try to let things heal" is an unfair one. I am involved. Ours was an important relationship [in] which I invested a majority of my free time for over a year. What I gave you wasn't just time, though. I gave you my emotional energy as well. I gave you my promise of monogamy which precluded me from making connections with other men with whom I might have built something real. I shared my life and my family with you. And so much more. No, Martin—I won't just go away. You have to face what you've done.

I believe if you find the goodness inside you that your mother helped cultivate you can find happiness again at some point with another woman, but that cannot happen by brushing me or what you've done under the rug.

From: Martin
Date: November 7, 2017 at 8:31:37 AM PST
To: Hayden
Subject: Re: What happened

Thank you for letting me know. I feel like my life is over. It's all my fault. Thank you for letting me know and I am sorry.

A little while later, Martin texted me to say that he was ready to tell the truth. I knew he knew I knew. I felt unstable and frightened. We planned to meet that afternoon at two o'clock at a nearby Starbucks.

I prayed that when he showed up, he would be the man I thought I knew. I prayed he would take ownership and reveal the truth to me in a loving, mature way.

I asked Dawni Rae to come with me and wait in the car until I needed her. I wanted Martin to have a chance to tell the unfiltered truth with just me. When I walked into Starbucks, he was there. He was the man I hoped for, well dressed and standing strong.

As we sat down, I asked him to tell me the truth. He hung his head and began to apologize. It was nothing that I hadn't already heard. He didn't tell me what happened but just kept going with the apology. I asked him for my keys.

"They're in my car," he said.

"Then go get them." I got out my phone and called Dawni Rae to ask her to come inside. After I hung up, I said, "I want her here. I know everything, Martin. Why? How could you do this to me?"

"I knew it was wrong. I thought about ending it, but I liked the attention and the feeling of someone wanting me. Every time I tried to stop, my ego and self-loathing convinced me to keep going. And then it just sort of fed on itself. The lies made me feel worse, and the worse I felt the more I needed you and her, to make me feel better. I lied to everybody, including myself."

I didn't say anything, but I was listening.

"I got scared around the time of my knee surgery," Martin continued. "The lies kept getting bigger. I sought counsel with Father Boyd, but even with him I stopped short of telling the truth. When you told me about your health scare, I wanted to tell you. I was afraid. When I got back from New Orleans and saw you, I knew how much I'd hurt you and how much I was letting you down. I felt even worse, but I hoped that somehow it would all go away. Somehow, I would snap back into being me. Somehow, I would be enough. I hated myself for what I had become."

Unworthiness is a dirty beast. I felt my heart soften. Just a little bit.

"Last week things came to a head. I wasn't sleeping, and I got really desperate and did some things that don't make sense. I apologize to you for all the lies and the embarrassment and stress I must've caused you. I wanted to make it all go away. I was so tired. I wanted to just go to sleep. I thought taking the coward's way out would be easier than the work I have ahead of me. I thought it would be easier not to live. You were my person and I hurt you."

I felt tears welling up in my eyes.

"This has nothing to do with you. These are my own demons! I'm not making excuses for the damage that I've caused you and my family. I stopped doing my work. I thought that I was going to be OK after I stopped drinking. I stopped going to counseling and stopped working through my fears. You've been nothing but good to me. I apologize from the bottom of my soul. I'm working to get the help I need to be the person I know is underneath this."

"Were you planning on leaving me?" I asked.

"I thought about it when I first met Hayden."

"Then why didn't you? Was it because of money, because I was financially supporting you? Did you use me for money?" He looked me in the eye.

"Yes," he said. "I used you." Another sucker punch.

"Our relationship is over. And you are fired, effective immediately." I looked at him, this man I loved. "I will miss you. It's time for you to go."

There was so much sadness and remorse in his eyes. I fell into Dawni Rae's arms and cried, and she held me as I watched him walk away. That was one of the most painful moments of my life. On November 7, 2017, we said goodbye.

The day after we broke up, I had a dream. I dreamed that I was being beaten to death by someone I trusted. An unassuming person whom no one would suspect. As I watched myself getting beaten, Martin walked over to my body. That's when I woke up.

Ever since I was a little girl, I've vowed that I would never go back to a man who abused me. That was one of my core values. The dream showed me that I had been abused, not physically but emotionally. I knew I could not go back. That was my truth.

The next day was excruciating. My nine-year relationship had completely disintegrated, and I had never felt such grief before. I kept wanting to reach for him. The very person who betrayed me was the person I wanted the most. You can't just turn off love. He was like a drug, and I was trying to go cold turkey. I needed one more hit to make me feel OK.

After the second day, I caved. I sent Martin a text. I told him the pain was unbearable. I opened the door to communication. We had a few brief text exchanges. But then I remembered my dream and I had to say a final goodbye. I wrote him this email:

> Dear Martin,
> I am so glad you were not successful in your attempt to take your life. This all would be even more painful if you had been. I am so grateful that you were able to show up on Tuesday as the man I thought I knew. You were honest. You stopped lying and owned what you did, confirmed the story and confronted the truth. We were able to talk things through in a mature way. That is the man that I love(d). This was what we had worked so hard in our relationship to be. I am happy we had one last chance to show the strength of our relationship, albeit in one of the most painful experiences of my entire life.
>
> All of this is almost too much to handle. It is so much to process and untangle. I am stunned and shocked that you were capable of all of this. It makes no sense to me. It is so out of alignment [with] the person I know you are. I want you to

know that I have so much compassion for you. I weep all day knowing that you felt so unworthy of my love that you could do something of this magnitude. It hurts my heart so much to know you are that wounded. Martin, I know you are not a bad person. I know that person I loved so deeply is not this. I will refuse to believe that our entire relationship was a sham. I know deep down that you did love me for most of our relationship. I feel the deep grief of losing my person and immense sorrow for you.

I really hope you are set free. I hope the burden of carrying these lies is now lifted and you can start to work to return to the person I know you are. It must have been so exhausting. Please know that I am in the process of forgiving you, but my heart already feels ready to. Because I know this is not about me. Yes, I was a willing participant in the separateness of our lives which made your double life possible. And yes, I also made the mistake of hiring you to work for me, which ultimately tore us apart and I believe was a huge part of your insecurity and feelings of unworthiness. But I loved you. You were enough for me. I gave my all to you and for you. I know this is your stuff and that is why I want to forgive you, so you can overcome some of your shame and move forward in your health.

This is the most pain I have ever felt. I have never had my heart shattered into pieces like this. It is hard to imagine life without you. It takes my breath away and makes my knees buckle. I am sick to my stomach.

I know I will come through this. I know you will too. I will hold our good memories close to my heart. There were many. I will not bury you or hide you away. I will not live from that place of hate or fear. I will miss you terribly in so many ways. My heart is so broken. This is a devastating loss for me. But the truth is here and I know I will eventually be set free too.

Martin, please know I love you. You are worthy of love. You are enough. I see you beyond these wounds. Letting go of you is going to be one of the hardest things I've ever had to do. But you are set free. Time to start new. I have no idea what my future holds but I am walking through the door to my next self.

There were several pleas from Martin in response to that email. Each time he came toward me, I got hooked back in. Finally, I told him I did not want any more contact with him for at least a month. I needed to start the process of acceptance.

I broke up with Martin on a Tuesday afternoon. Wednesday at noon I taught a yoga class. Even in my grief, I vowed to show up and let myself be seen. Tears rolled down my face and my voice shook as I taught. My students were used to seeing me as a pillar of strength and inspiration, but I was broken. I did my best, which was all I could do.

I spent the next several weeks feeling the grief. I had never cried so much in my life. I would go in and teach yoga, then, after each class, I would cry. At home and in the car, Alexis would sit with me and let me cry. "Just feel it," she'd say. "Take your time."

Even in that dark hour, I was so proud of her. At one time she'd been afraid to feel, and now, here she was, encouraging me to do so. She was strong, even in her own grief. She lost a friend, too, someone she loved and admired. She was very clear with me that I should never go back to him. Though she was experiencing her own loss, she knew the right answer.

I also spent a lot of time telling my friends and family the story. It was exhausting but helpful. It kept me aligned with my truth. People rallied behind me. It was no coincidence that the same women who'd come running to my side during my breast cancer scare showed up for me again.

Thanksgiving was right around the corner, and I knew the holiday was going to be tough. So I invited those same women to come over for a Friendsgiving. It was spontaneous and last minute, but Dawni Rae, Karina, Gail, Audrey, and Sarah came without question. Their partners came along too. And of course, my beautiful daughter and her best friend Alia Joy were there.

That night, I stood at the head of the table in my broken vulnerability and expressed my deep gratitude for those women. They were my gladiator warrior goddesses. They stood by me and were so strong and ready to fight for me. They didn't just show up that night, but every day, whether it was with a text or phone call, a dinner out or happy hour, or a run in the rain—they were there every step of the way. I'd asked for this *kula,* this community, and they were there right when I needed them.

My family was grieving too. My dad lost a son and his side of the family lost a man they really loved and cared for. Everyone was in shock. But, as during my divorce, my dad never wavered in his love or allegiance to me. He stayed by my side and said goodbye to his son. He made me feel so loved and seen.

At the studio, I showed up and did my best. I was raw, vulnerable, and transparent about what was happening to me.

The support was overwhelming. Those communities I had cared for and nurtured so long were now holding me up.

The grief fueled my teaching and touched many people. In fact, one day after yoga class, a student stopped me on the street near the studio.

"I never listen to the message," he said. "I really only come for the workout. But what you shared touched my heart. I'm going through a breakup, too, and now I know that I'm not alone. Thank you."

I'd been renting an Airbnb over the past year in White Rock, British Columbia, taking solo weeklong writing retreats to write this book. A month after the breakup, I went to the studio to teach a class before going up for another retreat to finish this book. This class, I decided, was going to be on heartbreak. My inspiration would be that pain is never permanent; the sensation subsides. We just need to be willing to feel it. Our spirits are stronger than our broken hearts.

I walked into the studio to discover that my Sunday four-thirty class was sold out. A few people even had to be turned away. That was a first for this class. I knew it was no coincidence. As I sat down at the front of the room, I gazed into the forty-five sets of compassionate eyes looking back at me and gave them my message. It was powerful. I was strong in my conviction and steady in my power. After class, I wept.

Earlier that day, I had gone down a rabbit hole. I started to wonder if Martin had cheated on me before, and, remembering all those pathological lies, asked myself, *What is this, person who I thought I knew, capable of?* Those queries bred fear, and by the time I drove up to Canada, I was in a full-blown panic. I barely slept that night.

The next day, I began writing this story, closing in on the end of the book. Being alone and writing in such detail, retracing every step toward the pain I now found myself in, took a huge toll on me. I had to stop.

I went for a run to try to "move it out." That didn't work. I went to a local café to be around people. It got worse. I then went to the store. The last time I'd been in that store was with him. I went to get coffee and the bottom shelf was lined with boxes of candy called Martin's. All of a sudden, I was paralyzed; I could not breathe. I'd never had a panic attack before but felt like I was on the verge of one.

I got back to the Airbnb and my sister Holly texted me. I called her back but got her voicemail. The moment I started to speak, I broke down. I could barely talk or breathe. I was in so much pain, so much fear. I called Karina for support. She told me she would call soon. I took a shower. With my hair wet, my body naked, I sobbed and wailed. Karina FaceTimed me and saw me at my most broken point. She just stayed with me. My heart tore open that day. I felt like it had literally broken. The emotions flooded out of me in the most visceral way. My wails were from the deepest part of me. Those wails were not only for him but also for all the times I had been abandoned.

During this process, I recognized something big. I realized that thinking of Martin as a "bad" person, a sick, pathological liar who had harmed me and could do so again, was easier than accepting the loss. I didn't need to know if he'd had other affairs. It didn't matter. I didn't need any more nails in the coffin. The coffin was already sealed shut. I wanted him to know how much pain I was in, but the truth was that didn't matter either. It was time to let it go. Time to accept loss through the lens of love.

Once I calmed down, I reread the email I'd written to him as my final goodbye. This place of love and compassion was where I would try to stand from then on. Even if that was the harder work. Even when we are wronged, we can stand with a face of love. Love is our *purpose*. Every. Single. One. Of. Us.

The truth was that I loved this man and he loved me. But the gap between us was too wide. Betrayal and truth cannot stand side by side. I lovingly released him to do his work and for me to do mine.

It was time for me to journey solo. It was the first time since I was sixteen that I had been on my own, totally and completely. I was ready.

On New Year's Eve, 2017, I wanted to say goodbye to the year in a way I had never done before. Every minute would be a demonstration of who I was now and what my purpose would be. Karina and I decided to go to a spiritual celebration at Bohemian Studios. Adrienne, who used to teach for me, owned the studio, and I felt safe to explore there. Instead of booze and balloons, I walked in to find tea, tarot cards, and stones of healing. We danced, then practiced yoga. After, we engaged in deep breath work that truly moved more trauma out of my body. We ended with a sound bath, which conjured deep gratitude for my life. I felt so aligned.

Karina and I continued our celebration at Golden Gardens Park. Under the full moon and cold sky, we built a fire, read poetry, and drank tea. At the stroke of midnight, we stripped off our clothes and plunged into the ocean as fireworks exploded overhead and moonlight beamed over our naked bodies. As I submerged in the water, I rinsed myself of my abandonment and overfunction issues. I said goodbye to my mother, to Martin, and to all the parts of me that no longer served me. I said hello to the next version of me. The person who was awake, whole, and seen. It was my own baptism of purpose.

Purpose Cycle Reflection Questions:

1. What would you do if you knew you would not fail and had the resources needed to do it? Better yet, what would you do even if you knew you would fail?

2. What makes you feel alive? What needs to die in order to be reborn?

3. What are your strengths? Remember, these are things that you are good at *and* enjoy doing.

4. What doors are you willing to walk through to see more doors open?

5. How do you view vulnerability? Are you willing to seek it out to create connection and reconciliation or find the truth?

6. Where do you carry shame? Are you willing to hunt it out in order to release it?

7. What are your core values that cannot be negotiated or rationalized in living your truth?

8. Are you willing to feel the greatest love but also the greatest pain?

Namaste

"The light in me sees and honors the light in you."

I started on the quest to write this book in the hope of inspiring people to be seen. The best way I know how is to lead by example and show up and let myself be seen. Through this process, I investigated every aspect of my life, sought vulnerability, hunted shame, and left no stone unturned in the search for truth, to see myself, to see love in its truest form. Like the lion in *The Wizard of Oz*, the courage was already within me. The truth was there too—I just had to see it.

No matter where this book goes, who reads it, who likes it or doesn't like it, it has served its purpose. I got to see more of myself, find the things in my life that were unresolved, and work to heal.

It is said that every cell in our bodies regenerates, and that we can transform into a new self every seven years. I'm forty-three at the time of this writing, so I have just started my seventh self. I have no idea where I will be in the next seven years. But I believe I will be born again with an even stronger sense of purpose. There is so much more to learn and see.

Through the Seen Cycles, from Primal to Struggle to Conform, then to Transform to Purpose, there is always more work to be done. If we break through Conform, we will Transform over and over again, deeper in our Purpose. If we allow ourselves to see and be seen, we will always be moving closer to our best life. Every mistake, every unconscious reaction, can serve as a wake-up call, a way to push us out of conformity, complacency, and dysfunction and toward our true selves and highest purposes.

Love is our greatest power. If we allow ourselves to see, we can learn to love that which we'd thought unlovable, feel compassion and tenderness for our wounds, and approach one another with universal, divine love. Love lets us forgive. Love lets us accept. Love lets us let go.

As with Russian nesting dolls, we have to unstack our outer layers to find the beauty right at the center of our hearts. It takes courage to see and be seen. But if we do, we find truth, freedom, and peace within. I know I did.

I'll be seeing you.

Acknowledgments

I am so grateful for my daughter Alexis. Thank you for being my biggest cheerleader. You are so brave and I burst with pride that I am your mother.

To my father, I am so honored to be your daughter. Thank you for choosing me when I needed you most. Thank you for teaching me your spiritual wisdom. Your spirit and love are truly divine.

Thank you to my best friend Dawni Rae Shaw, my constant source of inspiration and support. The decades of our friendship are so precious to me. I am so grateful for you.

To Karina Brossmann, deepest love and gratitude for your love. You helped me find my voice and taught me how to play again.

Higgins clan, you are the definition of compassion. I am so grateful to call you my family.

To my editing team, in particular, Anna Katz and Alexander Rigby, thank you for helping me tell my story and for your guidance and perspective.

To my yoga communities, hauteyoga Queen Anne and shefayoga Roosevelt, you are one of my greatest treasures. Thank you for showing up and being a part of the vision. I am so grateful for you.

To my teaching and front desk staff, I am so grateful for your loyalty, support, authenticity, and friendship. You are my family. I love you.

Thank you to my teachers who have inspired me to be a better teacher: Brene Brown, Sadie Nardini, Jennifer Pastiloff, Meghan Currie, Ashley Turner, Mastin Kipp, and Seane Corn.

Big love to Lululemon, especially those at the University Village store in Seattle, for fostering my leadership, supporting my vision, and pushing me to go after my big hairy audacious goals.

To my friends and family who supported me along the way: Heather Binckley, Maureen Higgins, Yvonne Leach, Gail Hudson, Jenniferlyn Chiemingo, Jill Spratt, Leah Adams, Audrey Sutton, Sarah Ilgenfritz, Casey Petersen, Michelle Chambers, Adrienne Rabena, Sean Dereck, Ginger Saunders, Mallory Monahan, Puja Telikicherla, Susan Grace, Brian Neville, Joey Ejeh, Hylke Faber, and Jeri and Amy Andrews.

About the Author

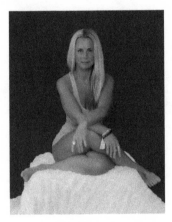

© hikepretty

Leah Zaccaria is a former certified public accountant with a master's in taxation turned yogi entrepreneur. She took her first yoga class in 2006 and later decided to marry her business expertise with her passion for yoga and opened her first studio, hauteyoga Queen Anne, in 2009, followed by shefayoga Roosevelt in 2013. She created Sendatsu Evolution in 2015, a teacher-training and leadership program that hosts several trainings, retreats, and workshops annually. She lives in Seattle with her daughter.